THE LIGHT WITHIN

LOIS M. RAMONDETTA, M.D., *und*

DEBORAH ROSE SILLS, PH.D.

THE LIGHT
WITHIN

———

The Extraordinary Friendship of a Doctor and Patient

Brought Together by Cancer

———

ωm

WILLIAM MORROW

An Imprint of HarperCollins*Publishers*

THE LIGHT WITHIN. Copyright © 2008 by Lois Ramondetta and Giles Gunn. All rights reserved. Printed in the United States of America. No part of this book may be used or reproduced in any manner whatsoever without written permission except in the case of brief quotations embodied in critical articles and reviews. For information address HarperCollins Publishers, 10 East 53rd Street, New York, NY 10022.

HarperCollins books may be purchased for educational, business, or sales promotional use. For information please write: Special Markets Department, HarperCollins Publishers, 10 East 53rd Street, New York, NY 10022.

FIRST EDITION

Designed by Kate Nichols

Library of Congress Cataloging-in-Publication Data has been applied for.

ISBN 978-0-06-135941-5

08 09 10 11 12   OV/RRD   10 9 8 7 6 5 4 3 2 1

In loving memory of

DEBORAH ROSE SILLS

BE NOT AFRAID

Comfort ye, comfort ye my people, saith your God.

Speak ye comfortably to Jerusalem, and cry unto her, that her
warfare is accomplished, that her iniquity is pardoned: for she
hath received of the Lord's hand double for all her sins.

The voice of him that crieth in the wilderness, Prepare ye the way of
the Lord, make straight in the desert a highway for our God.

Every valley shall be exalted, and every mountain and hill shall be
made low: and the crooked shall be made straight, and the rough
places plain:

And the glory of the Lord shall be revealed, and all flesh shall see it
together: for the mouth of the Lord hath spoken it.

The voice said, Cry. And he said, What shall I cry? All flesh is grass,
and all the goodliness thereof is as the flower of the field:

The grass withereth, the flower fadeth: because the spirit of the Lord
bloweth upon it: surely the people [is] grass.

The grass withereth, the flower fadeth: but the word of our God shall
stand for ever.

—Isaiah 40:1-9 (King James Version)

A cup of tea is a joy forever

—Deborah Rose Sills

CONTENTS

Preface *xiii*

1. The Patient *1*

2. The Doctor *15*

3. Leaving Kansas *31*

4. The Great Equalizer *59*

5. The Art of Dying *95*

6. Pas de Deux in Paris *123*

7. Spirituality and Cancer *145*

8. The Interview *171*

9. The Great Unknown *191*

10. The Distinguished Thing *201*

Afterword *by Giles Gunn* *229*

Appendix: *The Interview* *235*

PREFACE

The relationship between a patient and his or her doctor has, by nature of its intimacy and subject, been of interest to readers for generations. In recent years, with changes in medical treatment and technology, the nature of this relationship has changed dramatically. Treatments have become more effective, choices more numerous, and perhaps most important, patients increasingly well informed about their options.

In cancer care, where we are often contemplating the prospect of death, the relationship between a doctor and her patient can become very intense. What's more, with more women entering the field of oncology, and with cancer patients living longer, there already appears to be a shift in the types of relationships that tend to occur between patients and oncologists. Perhaps it is the recognition of the equality between women, the shared challenge of balancing work and family—something we all understand. Or perhaps it is merely the nature of women and friendship, so that even as doctors and patients we can share laughter, secrets, accomplishments, and open discussions about our hopes and fears.

This book is about one such relationship, and it is by and about the two women who shared it. Deborah Sills was a professor of religion, who was diagnosed with Stage III ovarian cancer; I was, and continue to be, a gynecologic oncologist who treats ovarian cancer. The idea of writing our story occurred to us when we realized how much personal satisfaction we gained from reflecting on the experiences our lives presented, especially in view of the fact that one of us was facing an early death. We worked separately at first, sending e-mails back and forth, sometimes leaving the manuscript for months at a time because our lives kept us so busy. But when we wrote, the process was relaxed and fun, and it brought us even closer together. We visited often, began traveling together, and even took time out from the manuscript to write for academic medical journals and to speak at medical conferences.

As the cancer progressed, we began to feel pressured to finish the book. The e-mails and writing retreats in Texas and California became more frequent, but over the final few months, as Deborah took a turn for the worse, the writing slowed again.

In the United States alone, there are more than ten million people living with cancer, and one and a half million others will be diagnosed with some form of the disease this year and in years to come. Cancer is not always fatal, of course, but ovarian cancer almost always is. Deb outlived the rates described in the actuary charts, and for almost a decade after diagnosis continued to teach and to enjoy the conversations of friends and family. She had an elaborate medical life, but she also enjoyed a rich social and academic life—a "big life," as she called it.

In March 2006, Deb decided that she was too exhausted to continue treatment. The only way for us to finish the book was to use a tape recorder and transcribe Deb's words, which I then read back to her for her editing. The completion of the book was immensely important to both of us for many different reasons, but primarily it was a way to immortalize our friendship.

I have never had a friend quite like Deborah Rose Sills, and I don't expect I ever will again.

Lois M. Ramondetta
August 2007
Houston, Texas

THE LIGHT WITHIN

1

THE PATIENT

I first met Deborah Rose Sills late one December evening in 1998. I was a fellow at the M. D. Anderson Cancer Center, in Houston, Texas, pursuing a career in gynecologic oncology, and she was a patient—a forty-nine-year-old woman with ovarian cancer.

I'd been on duty since 5:30 that morning, and at about ten o'clock—almost fifteen hours later—I finally made it back to my second home, a cramped hospital call room I shared with the rest of the trainees in my department. I'd reviewed my "To Do" list, collapsed onto the room's tiny bed, and drifted off to sleep, but I was roused a short time later by the insistent buzzing of my pager. I reached for the phone, none too happy, and dialed the nurses' station.

"It's Dr. Ramondetta," I said. "What's up?"

"The patient in room 710 won't drink her GoLYTELY," the nurse said.

I found this pretty irritating. I'm a New Jersey girl, only recently transplanted to Texas, and definitely am not as laid back as the natives. I didn't appreciate being robbed of sleep by a patient who seemed to have no regard for authority. To compound matters, she was my chairman's patient, and the political component only upset me further.

When I walked into her room, my arms crossed to show my displeasure, I met a woman who greeted me with equal obstinacy: Her hands were on her hips, and she stared at me, ready to do battle.

"So," I said, looking into her lively, defiant eyes. "I hear you won't drink your laxative."

"That's right," she replied, not blinking.

Deb's husband, Giles Gunn, a gentle-looking but slightly intimidating figure, was standing beside her. He seemed curious about the direction in which our stubbornness would take us, but I knew that this late-night summons could have only one possible ending: My chairman's patient was going to be prepared for surgery, whether she liked it or not.

"That's going to be a problem," I said, trying to keep my voice level and patient. "You have a small bowel obstruction that requires surgical intervention, and you are due in the operating room tomorrow morning. If you don't drink your GoLYTELY, there's not going to be any surgery."

"I haven't eaten anything in two weeks," she said. "I'm already empty."

"I know that's what you think, but we need to clean you out completely," I said. "Otherwise, there's a risk of spillage and infection."

"There's nothing to spill," she said, getting angry. "I've been throwing up for weeks."

"Deb," Giles said gently. "There's no reason to get upset."

She didn't answer. She just stared at me, waiting for my next move.

"Look," I said. "I can pour the stuff over ginger ale or put it on ice—it might taste a little better that way—but that's about all I can do. If you don't drink it, there won't be any surgery."

She looked at Giles, then back at me. She was still angry, but she knew she was fighting a losing battle. "Okay," she said. "I'll try."

"Thank you," I said. "That's all I ask."

The next morning she was taken to the operating room as planned. Since I was the physician at the bottom of the medical team hierarchy, it was my job to make the first incision, and I used a scalpel to open her abdominal cavity—all the way from her umbilicus to her pubic bone. I was relieved to see no visible cancer, the usual cause of bowel blockage in these cases, but her small intestine was matted with adhesions. The surgery was long and tedious—lasting over six hours in total. The team went from stricture to stricture, releasing each adhesion by sliding the scalpel along the outside of the bowel, as if scaling a fish. At each point of release, we advanced a few centimeters, until at long last we reached the end of the small intestine. With the job done, and with all of us feeling that it had been a success, Deb was sewn up and wheeled into the recovery room.

The following morning, as I did every morning, I made the rounds of all the patients on the gynecologic service. I usually started at 5:30 A.M., waking the patients, collecting vital data, and hurried to get done by six. I quickly learned that Deb needed to be left for last on morning rounds, otherwise I wouldn't have time to see the rest of the patients.

I will never forget how she looked in the morning. If she was awake, she would yawn and stretch her arms wide, as if trying to embrace the day, and she always greeted me with great vigor: "Good morning, Dr. Lois!" If she was asleep, I'd wake her with a gentle touch, and she'd open her eyes and smile broadly, waking with a loud "Hello!"

"How are you feeling?" I'd ask.

"I feel great!" she'd say, so full of energy she seemed lit from within.

Truthfully, it was hard for me to imagine anyone in her position feeling great. She had intravenous tubes in her arms, a nasogastric tube in her nose, and another tube protruding through the skin of her abdomen. The latter two were hooked to suction canisters on the wall. Despite it all, she was beaming.

"How can you feel great?" I asked, smiling. Her joy was contagious.

"Well, I've been told I have no cancer," she said. "And there's the possibility of eating again."

At that point, I knew very little about Deborah Rose Sills. I knew she was a professor of religion from Santa Barbara, California; that she was married and had two kids; and that she had been diagnosed with ovarian cancer the previous year. What I did not know then is that she and I were about to embark on one of the most remarkable relationships of my life.

I had come to the largest cancer hospital in the United States [Deb wrote] because I had not been able to eat for about two months. I had been diagnosed with Stage III ovarian cancer more than a year earlier and had undergone the standard therapies. After the requisite hysterectomy in October 1997, I had been given six rounds of chemotherapy that involved a relatively new drug, paclitaxel (Taxol), and an older drug, cisplatin. Cisplatin, in this instance, was delivered directly into my abdominal cavity through what is called, in the trade, an intraperitoneal catheter. My veins were never really very good, and, early on, my Santa Barbara oncologist, Dr. Margaret Sun, had ordered a Port-a-Cath inserted in my chest in order to receive the Taxol. The combination of the two drugs, and the cancer itself, made me very, very sick. I didn't know one could feel this badly and not die.

Every three weeks, for several months, I would spend the entire day at the cancer clinic, getting intravenous liquids to keep me hydrated or more accurately, to keep me standing. The clinic looked much like a furniture showroom. Naugahyde BarcaLoungers lined the walls, and if one was able to ignore the IV poles and the general debilitation of those occupying the chairs, one could imagine oneself thinking about redecoration and renovation. There was a surprising banality to the whole thing.

Generally, people don't get into trouble at the clinic while taking therapy. The trouble happens later, when one is home, alone, and it can involve a terrible fever, vomiting, diarrhea, and unimaginable fatigue.

I have always enjoyed spending a good deal of time alone, with music or a book or an old movie. I was six before my brother was born, have always managed to entertain myself satisfactorily, and, as an academic, I am habituated to sitting by myself and working things out. But I didn't sign up for the drama that unfolded in the days and weeks ahead.

Honestly, the effect of chemotherapy is something you watch without really understanding. During the months of nausea, I would sit outside our house with our two ranch dogs, wondering how long I could hold on, or even why I was holding on. I felt like a character in a Samuel Beckett play: "I can't go on. I must go on." All I could do was wait it out. Sometimes sleep felt as if I might die in it, giving way to forces of the body.

At one point, shortly after the chemotherapy began, I had asked my daughter, Abby, to cut off my hair as a preemptive strike, getting it before it fell out, and I went out and bought a wig. But even after my hair did fall out, I never wore the wig. Being bald seemed the least of my worries. I was under a kind of house arrest. During flu season, I could not go to movies or concerts, and if I did I wore a mask. I also wore a pair of dark sunglasses to manage the stares. It was my very own chador, minus the drape.

How illness changes your life!

I had led a life before illness that was heavily scheduled and that allowed for very little time for me. Nine years before my diagnosis, the family—Giles, Adam, Abby, and me—had moved to the Santa Ynez Valley from Santa Barbara. We lived on a small ranch that was a two-hour drive to my work at California Lutheran University, in Thousand Oaks, California. I was required to be on campus four days a week, and I had to leave the house by 6:00 a.m. to get to my first class, which started at eight. I could never seem to catch up. I was always late or unprepared.

Still, this was my life, and one looks for balance between what one might want to do and what is required of them. I believe I lived the required life. I kept the house running, loved my family and kids, managed to get tenure, went to the gym, and even danced a little. This is the drama of late twentieth-century American professional women. I had a job for which I had trained a full eight years. I had a wonderful husband, whom I managed to marry even when, as my father reminded me, I was "no spring chicken." Even more miraculously, I had managed to conceive and deliver a healthy and beautiful baby girl when I was thirty-five. But I was always tired, and often sick, and even, at times, inexplicably unhappy—so much so that on the drive to work I would occasionally cry for a full hour.

Then the cancer was discovered, and I really had something to cry about.

After six rounds of chemotherapy, I entered what I called the "Remission Society," but six months later, during another CA125 blood test—the test that serves as a tumor marker for cancer—I was told that the cancer seemed to have returned. Before long, I couldn't eat without experiencing terrible intestinal pain, and I was admitted to a Santa Barbara hospital.

The doctor there told me that the news would probably not be good—he felt it "in his bones"—and scheduled me for abdominal surgery. As they were preparing to wheel me out of my room into the operating room, my husband stopped them. "Don't you move this bed another inch," he said. Within hours, we were making plans to return to the M. D. Anderson Cancer Center, which I'd visited before during my initial chemotherapy regimen.

The night before the inevitable abdominal surgery, when I refused to drink my GoLYTELY, Dr. Lois showed up, looking combative with her arms crossed, and made herself perfectly clear: "If you don't drink your GoLYTELY, there's not going to be any surgery."

I made no distinctions among fellows, attending physicians, and physician chairpersons, but this one—whoever she was and wherever she fit into the hierarchy—was clearly very tough. Still, in retrospect, that first encounter was a win for both of us.

Seeing her the morning after surgery, I forgot all about our standoff the night before. I was simply grateful that no evidence of cancer had been found, and that the surgeons had been able to remove the bowel obstructions that had given me so much trouble over the last several months. I only learned later that Dr. Lois had opened me up and been part of the surgical team, and that she had peered at the very insides of her "difficult" patient.

How did Dr. Lois and I go from being a patient and physician at odds with each other one night to two women who were inter-

ested in what the other had to say? It could have been drugs, but there was something more—much more.

What I remember most clearly about this period of recovery was, to use the words of Ram Dass, "Being here now." I was completely in the present moment. It took up the whole of my imagination. I was focused solely on what was before me, working, if that word applied, to meet the requirements set down by my extraordinary nurses, who—from the very beginning of my recovery—demanded my full, emotional engagement. So, yes—I was in the present.

I remained in the hospital for two more weeks. The days started early, and I soon fell into the rhythm of hospital life, but what I most looked forward to were the mornings—to seeing Dr. Lois. She would wake me up before 6:00 A.M., check the various incisions and the tubing that protruded from my tummy, and ask how I was doing. Once we got the medical questions out of the way, the real conversations would begin, and I knew almost immediately that this was a woman I wanted to get to know.

One often thinks of the narrow circle that defines a life, and I found myself thinking about it then. At the university, I spent the day with academics, and at the ranch I associated with mothers like myself—women who had children in grammar school, our common bond. There were wonderful people in both groups, to be sure, but those relationships did not capture my imagination, and I lived every day with a hunger for more. I think part of the problem was that my friends looked too much like me, making it impossible to break out of that narrow circle. Or maybe it was something else entirely: my punishing schedule, driving six hundred miles a week, living a professional academic life, running a household, loving my husband and my two kids, entertaining from time to time, etc. I'm not sure what it was, exactly. All I know is that I felt then, as I do now writing this, that I never seemed to have enough time for the pleasures of living, and for musing upon the wonders of friendship and the accomplishments of others.

But Dr. Lois was a revelation—and an opportunity. Fast talking, beautiful, funny, and smart, she had studied both biology and religion at Emory University, in Atlanta. She remained interested in all things religious and seemed sure of a connection between healing the body and healing the spirit.

On her morning visits to my room, I inevitably wanted her to stay longer than she could or did. Her visits had a kind of intimate character to them. I knew she had other patients to assess, some of them in need of far more medical attention than me, but I wanted her to myself. I wanted to know everything about her. Who she was. Where she lived. How she had come to choose this daunting profession.

Every morning when I walked into Deb's room, I was curious and excited about what I would find, and about what she would have to tell me.

"Are you familiar with the writings of Ram Dass?" she asked me once in those early days. "It's about understanding life in its small moments. It's about learning how to think about where you are, not about where you've been or where you're going."

"How does one do that?"

"I'm not sure how others do it," she said, "but I have no choice. I finally understand that I can't live in a future that might not be there for me."

Deb was often physically cold—a combination of the cancer and the chemotherapy—and she had a collection of beautiful scarves and brightly colored hats that added color to her photogenic face. She showed me pictures of herself before she became ill, and she was beautiful then, too, but in those pictures I did not see the same love for life that radiated from the Deb I was beginning to know.

"You look more—I don't know," I said, faltering, "more *excited* now than you do in these pictures."

"You think so?" she said, peering up at me through her round, bright-red glasses, then glancing back at the photographs.

"I see so much energy in you," I said. "I don't know how else to explain it."

"The French have a phrase for that," she said. "Élan vital."

Yes! That was it precisely. Élan vital, vital force. It seemed to come off of her in waves.

"I'm curious about your work," she said. "How does one go about becoming a gynecological oncologist?"

"Can we talk about this on my next visit?" I said, glancing at my watch. "I really have to go now."

"You know, Lois," Deb said, her bright eyes twinkling. "I think I like you. I think I like you a lot."

I liked the fact that this was the only version of me that [Lois Ramondetta] knew. I can divide my life into stages to one degree or another, as perhaps all of us can. In my case, it was life B.C.— Before Cancer—and, now, A.D.—to use the Christian appellation "in the year of the Lord." If it is a recognition of grace at work in the world, I am happy to use it—even as a nice Jewish girl.

Some friends, I soon discovered, are better at cancer than others. For many, the fear of cancer and the specter of it in someone close is absolutely overwhelming. It invokes a personal terror that has very little to do with the person who is ill. It is the standard mantra—There but for the grace of God go I. Your friends ask you, "How are you managing the news?" "How does it feel to be bald?" "Are you in pain?" These questions are basically rhetorical. I remember being asked by one friend, "How are you feeling?" I told her I was fine, but she asked again. "How are you really?" What she wanted was a demonstration of my despair, a confirmation that it was as bad a business as she had feared, and it was, believe me, but I wouldn't give it to her.

Since my diagnosis, I have divested myself of many friends, some of long standing, who knew me B.C. And I have done this because in their eyes I will always be in an altered state—I will always be sick. And sickness can be terrifying. Sickness makes you think about the unthinkable.

With the people I have met since beginning this cancer drama, however, I am what they see before them. There is no other self, a self who might have been or who once was. There is just me. And, yes, I'm sick.

I had my family, of course—and one does not divest one's self of family. There was my son, Adam—Giles's son, really, from his first marriage—struggling to figure out how to communicate with me, what to say that might make me feel better, or to make himself feel better. And there was my teenaged daughter, Abby, who had been having a difficult enough adolescence B.C., and now found her life problems seriously compounded by my illness.

And of course there was Giles, my husband, who had also been redefined by my cancer—who had become, above all else, Giles the Caregiver. The fact that he was an internationally acclaimed author, an expert on globalization, and a professor of international studies at the University of California, Santa Barbara—none of that seemed to matter now. He was no longer Giles the Stellar Conversationalist, or Giles the Storyteller, or Giles the Recovering Motorcycle Aficionado. He had become Giles Gunn, the Professor with the Very Sick Wife.

He was there from the beginning, of course; steadfast, a pillar. He had a front-row seat in the early stages, after my hysterectomy but before the chemotherapy, when I began a psychic fall. This downturn began less than a week after that first surgery, while I was still recovering—while I was still trying to get my mind around what had just happened to my life—when my dear friend Walter Capps, a former teacher, a professor of religious studies, and a California congressman, died unexpectedly. I was brought to an abyss, an imaginary world that unraveled first with my own death, then with that of my dear husband. I imagined that our daughter Abby, then only thirteen, would be placed in a nightmarish orphanage, an experience from which she would never recover, and that our son, Adam, would roam the world, lost forever. Life unraveled in a hurry. Unimaginable terror filled my nights and most of my days. Walter's death signaled the triumph of darkness over the forces of light.

Giles saw me through that terrible period. He spoke to me with great affection and with a good deal of wisdom. "If fear wins when one is in the world, then cancer wins," he said. He was right. Death will take us all, but the real drama lies between one's terror of loss and the possibilities of the present. We are all frightened creatures. "Gird up your loins," as the Hebrew prophet Amos might have said, and get on with it.

2

THE DOCTOR

When I was in medical school, most of my friends were out in the world, making money, marrying, and having children. When I would complain, dreaming of the "neighbor's green grass," my father would say to me, "Lois, this is your life."

The goal was to keep me focused, and the message was simple: "You're on the home stretch. Everything you think you want can wait."

Even when I was in grade school, my father had devised a system of rewards: "You get three dollars for an A, two dollars for a B, and nothing for a C—because that's just average. And if you get anything less than a C, you're paying me."

He expected a lot from himself and from his family. "Every human being should be trying to make the world a better place," he used to say. "That's what it's all about: making a real contribution."

I was always urged to dig deeper, to reach for things that mattered, and to weigh my options carefully. The future was serious business. Normal life would come along in due course.

From the very start, even as a child of nine and ten, I was encouraged to think about college, and to wait on marriage and children. "There will be plenty of time for that later," my mother used to say. She was twenty-three when she had me, the first of two daughters, and I don't think she regretted it for a moment, but if you'd asked her, and asked my father, they might have said that the weight of family responsibility had kept both of them from living the life they had imagined.

For a time, I thought about becoming a teacher like my mother, but my father strongly encouraged me to consider a career in engineering or medicine. The straight path toward the "sure" future was emphasized, and as long as I followed that path my family would do what it could to support me.

Ironically, our family seemed to be guided by utmost practicality—even a degree of fear. But what did we have to be afraid of? There had been no physical sickness, no addictions, no cancer, and no prolonged deaths. Then again, perhaps the thinking was that we had been *too* lucky, and our luck was certain to run out. We need to save money, prepare for the future, limit excess, and learn that one needed to work for everything.

"'*You can't always get what you waaant*,'" my mother used to say, singing that old Rolling Stones song, but I was taught that if we tried, we'd get what we needed.

In college, I started to meet people who seemed to have had less structured and less predictable lives, which struck me as somehow being far more interesting. Of course, that could have just been me: I'm naturally curious about people, and I'm always trying to figure out what makes them tick.

By the time I got to Emory University, still looking for answers, I decided to major in religion. I studied Judeo-Christian basics and went so far as to be bat mitzvah'd, but I also participated in the chaplaincy program. The influence from my family was strong, though, so just to make sure I had all the bases covered, I also decided to fulfill my medical school requirements by doing a second major in biology.

Through the chaplaincy program, I found myself working in area hospitals, trying to comfort people who were facing death. It was an incredible experience. In sitting with them, and talking to them, I was being forced to come to terms with my own mortality. I looked for answers in books like *The Road Less Traveled* and *Good Grief*; nothing satisfied me, but I kept looking.

I also worked with Alzheimer's patients, and was terrified by what I saw—terrified by the notion that someone could forget who they were. I imagined it as a sort of death-in-life: *The people they had once been no longer existed*.

I would think about my own death, of course, or, in the case of Alzheimer's, try to imagine what it would be like to look in a mirror and find a stranger staring back at me. I took classes in ethics, world religions, even New Age religions; despite all this, the questions that had plagued me since about the age of twelve remained largely unanswered.

I also realized, probably as a result of these explorations, that I'd lived a very cautious, structured life, and I found myself hungering for adventure. I still wanted to go to medical school, mostly because I thought I could make a genuine contribution as a doctor, but I also considered taking a little time to join the Peace Corps, say, or to go to India to work with Mother Teresa.

"Absolutely not," my father said when I brought it up. "We are happy to help pay for medical school, but only if you go now. If you want to take time off, I can't promise we'll help."

I'm not sure I thought this was reasonable, but I didn't argue. Since most of my fellow students were going into massive debt to get their degrees, I felt very lucky that my parents were willing to foot some of the bill at all.

During my first year of medical school, at the University of Medicine and Dentistry, in New Brunswick, New Jersey, I was diagnosed with an abnormal PAP smear. It turned out to be nothing, but the examination experience itself was life altering. My doctor, who was male, ordered me to put my feet in the stirrups and then proceeded to examine me with a surprising degree of insensitivity. It was humiliating and painful, and I decided, consciously or not, that if I ever became a doctor I would never make that same mistake—that I would go out of my way to try to make my patients feel empowered.

Much later, while working with terminal patients as an obstetrics and gynecology resident, I began to see my future as a physician somewhat more clearly. I still wondered all the big *why*s that had never been answered in childhood or college: *Why did bad things happen to these people?* and *How will I handle my own mortality?* I began to really think about some of my patients, and even wrote stories about them, as if somehow that might help me figure things out. I wanted answers, and I wanted to dig deep, and during this period it occurred to me that oncology would put me close to "the edge"—close to the answers. Suddenly gynecologic oncology seemed like the right fit.

Before long, I became very involved with some of my patients, sitting at their bedsides, talking to them, holding their hands, letting them speak about their fears. I found myself becoming—in the parlance of the medical field—*radically empathic*. This expression speaks to both morality and philosophy. The idea, for a doctor, is to show empathy and compassion, but not to the point where you almost feel as if you're *becoming* the patient. It is too overwhelming, and doesn't make for sound medical decisions. A doctor need not be removed and uninvolved, but a little distance keeps emotion at bay, and too much emotion tends to cloud one's thinking.

Once, during my first year, when one of my patients was well enough to leave the hospital, she asked me if I would have dinner with her. "I'm sorry," I said. "I'm busy." And I *was* busy, but that's not why I declined the invitation; I declined because I wasn't sure it was *appropriate*. Or maybe I was simply trying to keep my life separate from theirs—to be as removed as the *real* doctors.

I felt a particularly strong bond with my female patients. I felt I could relate to them completely. I could identify with their concerns, their worries, and their insecurities, and as a result I was more confident about my ability to help them. It was exciting. Medical school had been the right choice for me, and gynecologic oncology the right field. One mystery was solved.

Despite the hectic pace of medical school, and the endless hours, I found time to get involved with one of my fellow students. His name was Ross, and he had blond hair, blue eyes, a bright smile, and great teeth. He was a man of eclectic tastes: camping, canoeing, playing Frisbee, even juggling. But he had little interest in spirituality—unless, of course, Grateful Dead guitarist Jerry Garcia counts as a spiritual entity.

By 1993, the two of us were at Jefferson University in Philadelphia, doing our respective residencies—Ross in emergency room medicine, me in gynecologic oncology—and we decided to get married. It was probably not the wisest decision. Being in medical school is very tough academically, but in many other ways it's a lot like being in college: None of it seemed like Real Life. Your parents—if you were lucky—were helping pay the bills, your hours were seriously regimented, and you lived at the beck and call of your superiors. In short, you did very little thinking for yourself. I know it bothered me that Ross had no interest in baring his soul in conversation— if I wanted to discuss my inner life and my inner demons, it would have to be with someone else—and I'm sure there were things about me that bothered him, but we hung in there. We were both overworked and sleep-deprived, and apparently too exhausted to do anything about our mutual dissatisfaction, and when I discovered I was pregnant about two years after we got married, my focus shifted from our faltering marriage to the excitement and promise of motherhood.

By this time Ross had a great job at a nearby hospital, but I was desperately hoping for a gynecologic oncology fellowship at M. D. Anderson Cancer Center in Houston. When I had applied, I had doubted that I would get one of the three coveted slots, but to my surprise word came back that I'd been accepted. When I broke the news to Ross, he was nothing less than supportive. Moving to Texas was not an easy decision for either of us since we'd be far from our families, but it was particularly tough on Ross. He would be leaving his friends at the hospital and a good job, and would be forced to start from scratch in a town where we knew absolutely no one.

Our daughter, Jessica, was born on February 2, 1997, and the following June the three of us moved to Houston to start life anew. We were excited—finding a house, furnishing it, settling in—but before long we were both caught up again in our demanding jobs, and life began to take its toll. The ninety-hour weeks, the lack of sleep, and the demands of parenthood were challenging enough, but ultimately it was the lack of intimacy that destroyed us. Ross and I were growing further and further apart, and neither of us had the energy to do anything about it.

The one constant in our lives was Elsa, the wonderful, even-tempered Ecuadorian woman who came along to help us take care of Jessica right after she turned one. I adored Elsa, and we couldn't have managed without her, but there were times that I was jealous of her relationship with my darling baby.

I would usually leave the house at 5:00 A.M., in what felt like the dead of night, while Jessica was still asleep. I often found myself crossing paths with Ross, who would just be getting back from his shift as an emergency room physician. On the way to work, I would miss Jessica so much that my heart would ache, but once I got to the hospital I had few moments to even think about her.

When I was on my way home at the end of the day or early the following morning, I would finally have time to think about Jessica again, and I would try to *not* think about the fact that our little world was falling apart. If it was after nine at night, I knew that Ross or Elsa might be in the living room with Jessica, trying to keep her awake so that I might at least see her for a short time, but sometimes, despite their best efforts, she'd be asleep when I got home. I'd go to bed absolutely shattered.

Weekends at the house were incredibly challenging. I would often arrive home on a Saturday or Sunday morning to find Ross preparing to leave for work. Since Elsa did not work on weekends, I was alone with Jessie. One morning, after a particularly grueling shift, I was so exhausted that it was all I could do to make the drive home, and I remember getting home to find Ross ready to leave for work.

"You've got to be kidding," I said. "You're leaving?"

"Yes," he said. "My shift starts at nine."

Jessica was just beginning to walk, so I had to watch her closely, and on more than one occasion, when I felt myself being overtaken by sleep, I would barricade the exits, block the electrical plugs, and pass out on the bed. I rationalized this by telling myself that plenty of toddlers went unsupervised, and that my daughter was such a clever little girl that she would manage to entertain herself for an hour or two. I still wince thinking about it.

On other occasions, alone with Jessica, I would put her into her car seat and we'd explore Houston until she fell asleep. I would then find a safe, suburban street, lock the doors, turn off the car, and go to sleep myself. When Jessie awoke, I would drive us to Starbucks, grab a coffee, and we'd go off to play in the nearest park. I loved those moments better than anything in the world, and I would feel completely renewed, capable of handling anything life could throw at me.

Work was tough, of course, but I never had any doubts about my chosen career. I remember sitting in the M. D. Anderson Cancer Center auditorium for oncology Grand Rounds one day, and writing a letter to a friend who was wondering if she, too, should specialize in gynecologic oncology. "The room is filled," I wrote. "The topic is head and neck cancers and advances in therapy. The initial speakers are well organized and clear and are flashing some interesting (gross) slides of tumors (for effect), and I am excited! All these people around me are working in all areas of cancer patient care and research, trying to cure cancer, or at least make a better life for people with cancer. If we remember the impact that cancer has on the lives of its victims and families, it is easy to understand what drew us to this field. It moves us and stimulates some of our deepest feelings about our loved ones and ourselves, and about how we want to see ourselves contributing to the world we live in. In fact, the desire to contribute can be so strong that sometimes I feel we should all be working frantically, around the clock, to find a piece of the cure."

Between July 1997 and June 1998, I was doing my so-called research year. I had always wanted to do something to advance the field, and research was certainly interesting enough, but if I had to choose between being locked up in a lab and sitting with a patient, well—there was no contest: I cherished human contact. Also, I was interested in the deeper mysteries of life, and I didn't think I would find any of those answers in a lab. And as I repeatedly told myself, there were plenty of doctors at M. D. Anderson who were better suited to that type of work. (And there are: One man in my department, for example, spends twelve to fourteen hours a day, sometimes seven days a week, focusing on basic research questions. I admire him, but I also know that I could never be that generous with my time, just as I wouldn't have been able to handle the solitude.) I needed my patients. I valued their lives and the intensity of their feelings, and I felt that my job was to be there for them during the cancer journey—and to try, in many situations, to make them as comfortable as possible as they embarked into the Great Unknown.

In late June, with my home life continuing to unravel, I began my first year as a clinical associate. If life at home was unpredictable, life in the hospital was all about routines. In the morning, I was obsessive about that first cup of coffee, which I usually savored on my way to work. Once in the hospital, I would do my rounds, write my reports, check the labs, then round again with a senior fellow. We would then race to the cafeteria and find something to munch on during the whirlwind 7:00 A.M. lecture, and by 7:15 I'd be in the OR or in the clinic, doing exams.

Surgeries sometimes went on for hours, and there was no such thing as excusing yourself to grab lunch. From time to time, the situation permitting, I'd sneak away for a quick slice of pizza. Sickness wasn't much of an excuse either, and I was okay with that—I don't remember ever staying home from school for illness, except for one severe episode of strep throat. Perhaps as a result, I am not terribly empathic about anything that isn't as serious as cancer. I guess I'm just lucky about my health. In medical school, I never had much time for exercising, reading, or cooking, and I had even less time for those pursuits at M. D. Anderson, but my body cooperated, and I soldiered on.

During my first clinical year of fellowship, the day ended anywhere between 6:00 P.M. and 9:00 P.M., but I still wasn't finished. Like a schoolchild, I had to be excused by my senior fellows—and we lower-level fellows weren't exactly a priority to them.

There are two levels of clinical fellows. I was still at the first level, and the second year fellow was actually "in charge." I prerounded, then presented to my senior fellow, who in turn communicated my findings to the attending physician. It was hard to feel confident in my decisions, especially when everyone seemed so focused on my mistakes, but I took solace from my close relationships with my patients, and that helped me bear the frustrations. Still, I'd be lying if I said it wasn't stressful. I wanted to be respected for my clinical decisions, and I wanted to *succeed*, but I was also thinking about the fact that my marriage was crumbling, and that my daughter was practically being raised by another woman.

Whenever I felt myself despairing, I would remember my father's words: *This is your life.* I had always been goal-oriented—it's a must for anyone who enters medicine—but now I wondered if perhaps I wasn't a little masochistic, too. In obstetrics you are bringing life into the world, and lots of joy. In gynecologic oncology, you are reflecting on life in the face of death every day—and yet hundreds of medical students were still drawn to the field. There were about thirty hospitals in the country that offered openings in this specialty, and each year they took only one fellow. M. D. Anderson, with a considerably larger department than most, took three.

If you're driven and accomplished enough to get into the program, which lasts three to four years, chances are good that you'll make it through to the end, but there are no guarantees. Fellows can be "excused" for any number of reasons. Sometimes they are told they don't have what it takes to succeed, and sometimes they find the work more depressing than they'd imagined. Those who leave, or are asked to leave, usually go during the first year. Those who stay become an "attending" at the end of the fellowship—a full-fledged doctor, officially—but the pressure continues unabated. You must publish in the medical journals to make your work known to your peers, and use that work to make your way up the ladder—first as an assistant professor, then as an associate, and, finally, as a full professor. It is primarily during the fellowship, however, in the day-to-day work, that you really start to prove yourself. Everyone is watching, everyone is judging, and you deal with it because you know they're only trying to make you a better doctor.

I was about halfway through my fellowship, still trying to understand the rhythm of the hospital, and the rhythm of my life, when I met Deb. It was December 1998. Things at the hospital were tough but manageable.

At home, however, things were getting harder. With my workload and schedule, with every passing day I felt like less and less of a mother. Every time I left for work in the morning, I still felt an almost physical tearing of my heart, and the pain stopped only when I walked into the hospital. Making my way along the corridors, I realized that in this place my problems seemed very small indeed. I was dealing with patients whose difficult questions put my own life into perspective. There was little time for self-pity, which felt, in any case, almost embarrassing to admit to. I saw this as a good thing.

Every four or five nights I was on call, as I'd been the night I met Deb. This required sleeping over at the hospital, doing morning rounds, and not getting back to the house till the following night. This period of my life is such a fog that it still feels like a dream. One of the few things I remember is the early-morning walks up and down the long, quiet hospital corridors, as I checked on my patients, many of whom were a tremendous source of inspiration. Every day, I was sitting with women who were facing almost certain death—*Amazing Women*, as I took to calling them—and I wanted to know absolutely everything about them. I would jot down some of the things they said on scraps of paper, and every day I'd fill my pockets with bits and pieces of our conversations. These women were just like the rest of us. They had hopes. They had fears. And they still had dreams.

On bad days, I would think back to what one of my attendings was always telling me: "Lois, you can only do what you can do." On good days, inspired by these Amazing Women, I would think, "If only I could be as courageous as they are! If only I could be more like them!" My little concerns were insignificant compared with the big picture.

I remember one sixty-year-old woman with recurrent ovarian cancer. Her stomach became constantly bloated with abdominal fluid, and one way to deal with this was through a "tap," also known as a paracentesis. The fluid would slowly drain into vacuum bottles, sometimes as much as four to six liters' worth, but she always walked out in a good mood. "Why do you always leave this place smiling?" I asked her.

"Well," she explained, "I can't eat with a belly full of fluid, and every time I leave here I go straight to my favorite restaurant and my favorite food—crab claws."

"Sounds delicious!" I said.

She smiled her big smile. "My mama used to say, 'Girl, you can get used to anything in this world. Hell, you can get used to *hanging* if you hang long enough!'"

Another patient was a real Texas cowgirl, a big-boned blonde in her early forties whose hospital room was decorated with photographs of her beloved horse. By the time I met her, she was near the end, and she knew it, but she didn't want to broach her death directly. "I saw a belt at the mall last week," she told me one day. "It cost several hundred dollars. You think I should buy it?"

"Absolutely," I replied.

On another occasion, she expressed interest in a pair of custom-made riding boots. "They take six months to make," she said. "What do you think?"

"I'm not sure about that," I told her as gently as I could, my heart breaking. She knew she was dying, and she was slowly coming to terms with it, but she could only face it in tiny increments.

There were moments of levity, too. Once, at the less upscale county hospital where I also worked, I was in a crowded examining room, separated from the neighboring bed by only a flimsy curtain. I was working on a new patient, and I told her, "I'm going to have to do the rectal now."

"Oh no you're not!" she shot back, and the women in the adjoining beds burst into laughter.

And there was depth, too. I had one patient, extremely ill, who always managed to smile when she saw me coming.

"How do you do it?" I asked her. "Where do you find the strength to be in such a good mood?"

"Honey," she said. "A year ago they told me I'd be dead in two weeks, and I'm still here, so, as far as I'm concerned, every day is a gift."

She was right: *Every day is a gift.*

3

LEAVING KANSAS

One of the first things I learned about Deb was how much she disliked to be defined by her illness, and how deeply it had affected her friendships. "I don't want to be seen as a sick person," she said. "And I don't want to be the site for these people to work out their own feelings about mortality."

Deb did not suffer fools lightly. She was a fiercely intelligent woman, and the fact that she liked my company made me feel good about myself. In light of the fact that my personal life was a shambles, her validation was doubly important to me.

I got to know her in three distinct steps: first, and very

briefly, as an ornery patient. Then as a woman with cancer. And, finally, as a friend.

I used to wonder if I was crossing some ethical line by allowing myself to become so close to her, and it worried me. But I looked at the situation as dispassionately as possible, and I could find nothing wrong with it. I didn't do any more or less for her than I did for any of my other patients—I did as much as I could for all of them. And I was friendly with many of the women under my care, though admittedly not at that level, nor with that intensity or that depth. Finally, I wasn't officially her doctor—that job fell to Dr. Robert Bouquet and Dr. David Goodman. I was *tending* to her, but I wasn't running the show.

Honestly, though, she was impossible to resist. And it went beyond charisma. There was something inside her that really pulled you in. I remember walking into the cafeteria and feeling her presence before I saw her. Then I looked, and sure enough—there she was, all the way across the room. She was wearing a bright red hat and a colorful scarf, and when she caught my eye she laughed out loud, giddy with joy. It made me giddy, too. She had a hearty, infectious laugh that seemed to travel great distances.

I joined her for a five-minute lunch. "So?" she said. "Got any good gossip?"

"Not a word," I said. "I haven't heard anything."

"Well, you see that doctor there?" she said in a furtive whisper, nodding in the man's direction. "I think he's sleeping with my pretty chemo nurse."

"No," I said. "He might be sleeping with the nurse in

admitting. Of course, he's married and has two kids, but that might not stop him."

"The nurse in admitting?"

"That's the one."

"I love dancing," she said. "I love ballet. I can't wait to go back to Santa Barbara and start dancing again." Then, abruptly: "Any improvement on the home front?"

"None," I said.

"What a pisser."

"Yes," I said, smiling despite it all. "What a pisser."

Everyone in the hospital seemed drawn to Deb. Doctors, nurses, even some of the cafeteria workers. She had energy and enthusiasm, and that big, hearty laugh that announced her presence, and she was honest in a way that was almost palpable. There was an underlying *truth* about the woman. Also, when Deb looked at you, she really looked at you. You felt like the center of the universe. She wasn't thinking about answering e-mails, or what her daughter was up to, or even her cancer—she was there, focused on you. She took pleasure in hearing people express themselves. She made everyone feel as if they were the Most Interesting Person on the Planet. Being in her presence was somehow *nourishing*.

Of course she didn't like everybody, and if you were one of the unlucky ones you felt it almost immediately. Deb wasn't mean about it, but she had a way of turning away, of losing her focus, and that, too, was palpable. It was as if she were saying, "I don't have much time left, so I have no time to waste, and I'm very sorry—I can't make room for you."

In effect, as she might have said, this worked to everyone's advantage. There was a level of honesty there that allowed no room for the small deceptions that most of us tolerate—and practice—as we make our way through the day. In short, Deb was not a fan of bullshit.

Deb often talked about living an "imaginative life." Reading, traveling, *hungering* for knowledge. She seemed to know a great deal about everything, and in the space of one conversation she might talk about everything from philosophy to a Disney character—from Plato to Pluto. That's what it was all about, she said: feeding the imagination; being open to anything and everything. Being *interested*. And she certainly was interested.

I remember talking to her at length about a lovely Hispanic woman on whom I had operated, and whom I felt I had failed. I had lain awake, ruminating over the surgery, wondering if I had done my best—or even if my best was good enough.

In that particular case, I had been forced to decide between bowel surgery or the insertion of a gastric tube and hospice placement. The former offered hope; the latter would be the beginning of a quick goodbye.

I really struggled over the decision. I reviewed her CT scan and saw much disease, but I believed that the surgery—an end colostomy, in which I would bypass the large tumor in her pelvis—might extend her life by a few months. When I opened her up, however, I had to rethink my plan. The amount of disease ruled out the easy colostomy I'd been hoping for, and even a gastric tube was impossible. I decided, partially motivated by my emotions and desire not to fail her, to go ahead and attempt the colostomy, and the procedure went as well as could be expected, but I knew it wouldn't be enough.

Every day I would look in on her, hoping for some improvement. She would lie there with a veil covering her head and her collection of Mother Mary faith cards arranged around on her pillow by her sister, who was always at her side. I felt awful, and I spoke to my colleagues about it, and the replies were always the same: "You can only do what you can do." "You're a great surgeon, Lois, you did your best." "You didn't give her the disease."

The morning I told Deb about this patient, she could see I was still in great turmoil.

"Let me understand this," she said, having heard the entire story "You took a lady to the OR who might have died a long, painful, bloated, nauseated death, and did your best to help her."

I managed a smile. Deb was right. I *had* done my best.

Days later, my patient became nauseated, indicating that she was blocked at yet another site. She died a few weeks later, and I still felt badly. If I looked at it logically, I had done nothing wrong. But this was emotional—and logic and emotion seldom mix.

"Lois," one of doctors told me. "You can't take credit for all the good, or you'll have to take credit for all the bad."

It helped a little, but even now, thinking back on it, the loss hurts. So many of them do.

. . .

That Christmas, not long after I met Deb, the nurses on her floor took part in the hospital's annual talent competition. They created a diorama based on James Cameron's film *Titanic,* but in their version the ship didn't sink.

Artistically and metaphorically, I saw what the nurses had done for both the staff and the patients, Deb wrote. *In their rendition, the tragedy of lost lives and lost love was reinterpreted and given another ending. It was no longer a tragedy that proved the inviolability of class distinctions and the hubris of the human enterprise to overcome nature. In this version, the* Titanic *arrives safely in New York Harbor, and the young lovers begin a new life together in America. They were challenging the standard ending in our ward—life cut short by fatal disease—and bringing the dead back to life. What if the* Titanic *didn't sink? What if the lovers lived together happily ever after? What if some of us got out of there alive?*

When I discussed this with the nurses, they asked if I would be good enough to put some of these thoughts in writing, which I did, and the project earned an honorable mention in a hospital-wide talent competition. A few days later, as a result of this unexpected victory, the nurses and I went off to have our photo taken with the hospital's president. En route, as I was making my way through the cafeteria, dragging my IV, I stopped to admire the extraordinary Christmas buffet that had been laid out for visiting dignitaries. I realized that I had not had a real meal for two solid months, since mid-October, and I don't remember being particu-

larly hungry—but I do remember the visual impact of so much beautiful food. Turkey, roast beef, vegetables, salads, desserts— everything lovingly arranged to catch the eye of those lunching with the president.

"Deb," I told myself. "You're not in Kansas anymore." Not in Kansas indeed. I was Dorothy, and I had stumbled into Oz. The world was alive with color, but I'd been living in black and white for so long that I'd forgotten what it looked like.

Suddenly I became aware of how far removed I'd become from what passes for normal life—the world of eating and sociability, of work and rest. I really was in the Kingdom of the Ill, and, in my case, the key to the kingdom was food. This experience is not peculiar to me, but part of the general experience of women with ovarian cancer. The inevitable march to starvation might begin with chemotherapy, or radiation, or scar tissue from surgery, or simply the cancer itself. I found myself thinking of Fran Lantz, a dear friend from Santa Barbara, who had herself been hospital- ized with ovarian cancer, and who told me one morning, near the end, exhausted, "I would really love a piece of roast beef." But of course this was wishful thinking. Meat is one of the first foods to go. When one does eat, one gets rice or cereal or cooked veggies—a return to childhood, but not in a happy sense.

After the picture-taking ceremony, I returned to my hospital room, still thinking of all that food—and fell into a very deep sleep. I was overcome by memories of my life before illness, and for the first time I think I finally understood, viscerally, the long- ings of the really hungry. Literature is full of such stories. Down and Out in Paris and London and Les Misérables have political *messages, but now I mostly remembered the descriptions of collective starvation. Even Somerset Maugham's* Of Human Bondage, *a book I had read as a teenager, expressed the anxiety of the poor and hungry hero. Up until that day, however, I had never fully understood the physical terror and human anxiety of not eating. I began to understand why, in Islamic Paradise, men are served the most magnificent dishes by seventy Muslim virgins. I began to see why Jesus turned the water into wine at the wedding at Cana, and why he made a feast for the multitudes when he delivered the Sermon on the Mount. Virtually all religious literature is full of food and images of tasting and eating. The Psalmist even wants to eat in "the presence of [his] enemies," at a table prepared by the Lord. I too wanted a meal, but I would have to wait.*

Two weeks later, the tubes were removed from my arm and from my nose and I was given a bowl of Jell-O. The following day, I was discharged to the Rotary House, a "holding hotel" across the street from the hospital. As I waited for my husband to return to Houston to take me home, I felt that I had been given back my life. After all, as the doctors themselves had told me only days after the surgeries, the biopsies were clear—there was no sign of cancer. "Thank you," I had said, bursting into tears. "My daughter is only fourteen years old. You have given her back to me. You have given me back my life."

What I didn't know, and perhaps didn't want to know, was that ovarian cancer has a terrible habit of recurring. As far as I was concerned, this cancer was survivable. As soon as I recovered from the surgery, I'd go back to my life B.C.—Before Cancer. I was in good spirits.

A few days later, when Dr. Lois came to visit with her daughter, Jessie, who was just three months shy of her second birthday, the world seemed full of promise and possibility.

The weekend after Deb was discharged, I took Jessica with me to visit her at Rotary House. It is across the street from the hospital, accessible through a sky bridge, and it looks like a pleasant, medium-priced hotel.

Seeing patients in their normal clothes after a long stay in the hospital always prompts reflection. Suddenly you are reminded that they are real people with real lives and their own style. It is also about how they want to be seen. Visiting Deb was important to me because I had already somehow entered her world at the bedside, but no matter how much I enjoyed our visits, there was always a part of them that was medically obligatory. I wanted her to know that I liked her and that I valued her as a person and, potentially as a friend; that she wasn't just a patient.

Deb seemed to radiate a special light that warmed me in a time of loneliness in my own life. I was surrounded by people like myself, medical school graduates and doctors, some of them in marriages that were as unhappy as my own, and most, like me, with little time to read, philosophize, and dream. Our worlds were filled with work, children, and daily routines. Deb was offering me much more.

It was a beautiful December day. Deb and I walked around the hotel grounds, talking, with Jessie trailing. Deb gave Jessica a tiny worn teddy bear that her own daughter, Abby, had given her when the cancer was first diagnosed. Deb said that it helped her recover from the surgery, but that she didn't need it anymore. The bear was very ragged and looked as if it had been through a lot, just as Deb had been, but Deb was a long way from defeat.

"This is what I've learned," she said. "You need to think about the impermanence of life every day. You have to get out of 'Kansas.'"

If you wanted to live with your head in the sand, she explained, you stayed in "Kansas." But if you wanted to evolve and grow, you left town—and you did this by grappling with the Big Questions. *Who am I? What does a life add up to? What happens after?*

"I do think about mortality every day," I said. "I don't have a choice."

It was true. Sometimes I felt so overwhelmed that I wanted to run away—wanted to be outdoors with my daughter, in the sunshine, feeling connected to life and to every living creature—not so *surrounded* by terminal diagnoses. This usually happened if I felt I had somehow failed one of my patients, if I'd found, for example, that nothing I could do or say would console them. I would tell myself that the next day would be better, and somehow, invariably, it was.

"I wish I could take one of your religion classes," I told Deb. "Maybe I could figure some of this out!"

I told her about one of my patients at the time, Helena Ramirez, a woman of sixty with so many bowel obstructions that surgery was no longer viable. She spoke no English, and usually I would communicate with her in broken Spanish. The day I broke the news, I'd brought someone along to help me translate. "Mrs. Ramirez," I said. "I'm sorry to tell you this, but we can't operate. There are too many obstructions. I'm sorry."

I waited for the translator to finish, and Mrs. Ramirez listened patiently, taking a moment to process the information. "I understand," she said, trying to be strong.

"I'm recommending that you consider hospice," I said.

Mrs. Ramirez began to cry, and I reached over and held her hand. "I'm sorry," I repeated. Behind me, the translator was also crying.

"It is okay," Mrs. Ramirez said. "I have three daughters, and all three of them are pearls, and I will wait for them in heaven."

I stayed with her for a time, doing my best to comfort her, and when I left the room I felt sad and hollowed out. I wrote a short note in her chart, summarizing our conversation, and thought back to an afternoon early in my fellowship, when I followed a faculty mentor into the surgical waiting room to give a family bad news about their mother. Nothing he said could soften the blow or stop the family's flood of tears.

When we left, I wondered how many of these talks I had in me. Five hundred? A thousand? Or, worse, how many hundreds of times would I be broaching the subject with one of my dying patients?

Many months later, I discussed these concerns with a palliative care doctor who told me: "Lois, sometimes the best thing you can do for a dying patient is to sit with them in silence. And that's often the hardest thing to do."

In due course, I discovered he was right. Figuring out how to talk to patients about death, and how to *listen*, is one of the toughest of the many tough situations we in cancer care are forced to deal with every day. At some point, all good oncologists will have the hoping-for-the-best-but-preparing-for-the-worst conversation. Careful planning can make it easier, but honesty and presence is more important. It is imperative for us, as doctors, to leave our personal issues at the door. We need to walk into that room and be completely focused on the patient. We need to sit next to them, at eye level, review what we've done and what we might still do, then talk to them about the most peaceful way to manage life in the face of death. We call this *making the patient DNR* (*D*o *N*ot *R*esuscitate). Some of us are good at it, some of us are not, and some doctors approach the subject with a discomfort bordering on terror. Perhaps theirs is a form of denial because it translates as defeat: You have to admit to the patient, and to yourself, that the battle has been lost. These doctors keep testing, poking, probing, medicating, because if they don't they are as much as admitting, to the patient and especially to themselves, that they are powerless—that there is nowhere else to go, nothing else to do. But when there's nothing else to do, why keep doing it?

With time, I began to get better at these talks. I began to see, for example, that these exchanges were not one-time summits, but give-and-take conversations. They required education, trust, and honesty, and—perhaps most important—a desire to really get to know the patient. Not really knowing a person results in either brutal honesty or total lack of it, so I made an effort to know as much about my patients as they were willing to share with me and, if our time was going to be very brief, to do so as quickly as possible. Mrs. Ramirez had come to us late in the game, and I was saddened because I never had an opportunity to get to know her as well as I would have liked. She was discharged two days after our talk, and she died three weeks later.

Not long afterward, I attended a lecture on physician wellness. It was delivered at the hospital by a professor of humanities at the University of Texas, and the crux of it was that we had to watch for burnout—that the weight of this collective sadness could creep up on us. The professor quoted from a Taoist poem, "The Woodcarver," by Chuang Tzu: "I am only a workman. / I have no secret. There is only this: / When I began to think about the work you commanded, / I guarded my spirit, did not expend it / on trifles that were not to the point."

The message was clear: When I had a job in front of me, when I was with a patient, I had to forget everything else. I had to focus fully on that patient. The world had been reduced to just two people, my patient and myself. Trifles were not to the point.

I would try to imagine what it was like for these dying women, what it must feel like to know that time is running out, and would give them the thing I had to offer: my undivided attention. When I wasn't at the hospital, however, my mind was everywhere. "I can't seem to focus on *any one thing*," I told Deb.

"That's what I've been trying to tell you," Deb said. "About being in the present."

Deb stayed into mid-December, recuperating, and I went to see her whenever I could. One night, shortly before she returned to Santa Barbara, we went to the home of one of the trainees and made Christmas cookies, and Deb played the violin for us. She was surprisingly good, but she laughed off our compliments. "I love playing," she said. "But I am very much an amateur."

This was not entirely accurate. Deb had played with the Los Angeles Youth Symphony, and had majored in music for the two years she spent at UCLA before transferring to the University of California, Santa Barbara. She had also been a member of the Brentwood Symphony Orchestra—so she was not exactly without talent.

At Christmas my parents came to visit, and we happily succumbed to the Catholic side of family tradition by sharing presents. We had a Christmas tree, too, with a handmade Star of David on top; that remains a tradition to this day.

One of Jessica's many gifts included one from a cousin—a little doll that lit up when she had a temperature. For reasons that were never clear, Jessica called her "Nancy," and she spent much of her time taking her temperature and giving her a bottle, and delighting at the way her nose and ears turned red when she had a fever. One afternoon, she decided to give

Nancy a bath; and Nancy stopped working, and her hair got so knotted up that she looked like a Rastafarian. Jessie didn't mind at all, though. She loved her as much as ever, with or without the glowing ears and the red nose.

Not long after, I went to my mailbox and found a gift from Deb. It was a book, *Fearless Girls, Wise Women, and Beloved Sisters: Heroines in Folktales from Around the World.* I think Deb was trying to pay me a compliment, and I certainly appreciated it, but she was the fearless one, not me. In the months ahead, I would come to believe more and more in the veracity of this statement, as Deb found herself struggling with an unexpected recurrence of cancer—and with the effects of the illness on her beautiful, adolescent daughter.

Before my cancer diagnosis I was a substantial middle-aged woman. About five foot six inches tall, I weighed between 135 and 140 pounds. I had a full head of brown curly hair and looked— at least in my memory—formidable. Leaving M. D. Anderson after abdominal surgery in December 1998, I weighed in at 113 pounds. I was skinny in a sick sort of way and had short curly gray hair. I had very little stamina and devoted the next six months to eating on a regular basis. The surgery was a success. I was eating oatmeal, baked potatoes, cooked veggies, and an occasional salad with tuna. My medical life involved monthly blood tests with Dr. Sun in Santa Barbara, and an occasional conversation with Dr. Robert Bouquet and Dr. David Goodman—my principal doctors at M. D. Anderson. I was able to stay in touch with Dr. Lois as she continued with her fellowship, and I repeatedly asked her to come visit us in California.

My recovery from abdominal surgery also involved my return to ballet. In fact, all I wanted to do after my initial diagnosis with ovarian cancer was to dance. I can't finally say why it was so important to me. I had danced casually as a kid and a teenager, but my mother's drunken afternoons had derailed my afternoon trips to Brown Gables Academy of Dance in Los Angeles. I didn't drive and she didn't want to. Yet ballet has always been alive in a distant place in my imagination.

I danced through college and then, with a great deal of commitment, through graduate school. Marriage and children brought an end to my adult ballet career. It is an urban activity that requires a level of cosmopolitan sophistication that was hard to come by in the Santa Ynez Valley, yet after my initial diagnosis, dance I did. I became a sort of middle-aged mascot to the professional ballet company in Santa Barbara, State Street Ballet. Its founder and artistic director, Rodney Gustafson, was a former principal dancer with American Ballet Theater, and together with his wife, Allison, also a dancer and not incidentally a professor of sociology, they created State Street Ballet and the Gustafson School of Dance.

I credit Rodney and Allison and the professional dancers of State Street Ballet with keeping me in the world. I would take class at least four times a week. I couldn't do the pliés and pirouettes that were once part of my repertoire, but I was alive.

That fall, the results of the CA125 blood test that Dr. Sun had been giving me monthly began to look "suspicious," as oncologists put it. What this can mean of course is that the cancer has recurred.

This is the main test for ovarian cancer. Apparently, in the early stages of cancer, it has as many false positives as false negatives. But once you've been diagnosed and are undergoing treatment, it is very reliable for tracking the changes. I could not believe it. I felt great. I was dancing almost daily with the State Street Ballet and could finish the class with my very own modified version of a grand jeté. I was eating, having sex with my husband, and fighting with my kids. It was normal life as far as I could tell.

A CT scan taken in Santa Barbara was reread in Houston and both Drs. Bouquet and Goodman saw a cancerous lymph node, a node the radiologist in Santa Barbara had overlooked. This discovery led to what is termed a "fine-needle biopsy" of the node, which in turn disclosed that the original ovarian disease had reappeared. My husband and daughter Abby were with me, and it was a sad business. Waiting for test results was part of my whole life, but at that point in my treatment it was full of terror and family drama. My then fifteen-year-old, confused by the dilemmas of adolescence, was overwhelmed by the prospect of having a dead mother sooner rather than later. She had been down this road once, and she didn't want to go down it again. Giles was just so sorry—sorry that I had to undergo this ordeal, sorry for the character of our lives together. And where was I? Abby's crying helped me move past myself and do a motherly thing—comfort my fearful child, hold her, and feel the warmth of her lovely teenaged body.

Dr. Bouquet suggested that I return for treatment and then enroll in a phase II clinical trial that M. D. Anderson was conducting under the guidance of Dr. Michelle Darling, a member of the Department of Blood and Bone Marrow Transplantation.

This clinical trial was designed for ovarian cancer patients who had recurrent disease, and it offered them the only possibility for cure that was currently available. It involved a preliminary course of standard chemotherapy—carboplatin and paclitaxel—and then a bone marrow transplant, an arduous chemotherapy drama that involves dying and being brought back to life. This must be done in the hospital and, as the social service staff of Dr. Darling pointed out, is not for everyone. Virtually all patients who undergo autologous bone marrow transplantation (BMT) with chemotherapy are accompanied by a friend or by a family member. This is not something one can do alone. It is both a physiological and a psychological undertaking. After thinking about it, and discussing it with Giles, I decided to go through with it.

Before I left for the seven-month BMT ordeal in Houston, I looked around for a therapist. I went to one woman who told me I needed to dress differently. I met with another who was so happy that I was going to die, and not her, that she cried when I told her I was not coming back. Ovarian cancer for women invariably provokes that old refrain: There but for the grace of God go I. *Perhaps cancers of all kinds do.*

Finally, I found a psychologist in Santa Barbara, a Freudian analyst, whom I saw for a short while at least once a week. I was full of rage and grief, and I had some accounts to settle. Both my parents were dead, and I had not spoken with my brother for fifteen years.

In his dark office off the main street of Santa Barbara, I tried to resolve these accounts as best I could. I tried to come to terms with disease, imperfect parents, personal failure, and the brev-

ity of human life. I did not do this alone. The analyst provided me the place and nudged me forward. I think I cried for about a month, and then there was the period when I was just alone and all I wanted was the company of our two ranch dogs, Oliver and Sheba. I was an unfriendly wife and an angry mother.

I have one other vivid and very painful memory from that period. I received an afternoon phone call from the Santa Barbara police department that informed me that Abby had been arrested for shoplifting at the local Long's Drugstore. Would I come down? Bald, masked, and wearing purple rubber gloves, I arrived at the drugstore, where I met Giles and the police officers. Abby was crying hysterically. I informed the officers that I was enrolled in a phase II clinical trial to treat ovarian cancer, and that I was expected shortly at M. D. Anderson in Houston, where the bone marrow transplant would be getting under way. The issue before us was simple: Would Abby be allowed to go to Houston with us or would she have to remain in Santa Barbara for trial? At that point, I crossed some sort of internal river. Despite all of our interventions, all the conversations, arguments, and worse, we could not manage to keep our daughter safe. I told Abby and I told the officers that it was now between "Abby and the law." I was actually beyond anger or disappointment. I was now just tired. I had been worn out, worn down by disease, by cancer treatment, and now finally by the daughter I loved so much. I turned my face away from her and put a good deal of psychic distance between us. This may be what all parents should eventually do anyway. The Dhammapada tells us that neither money nor our children are actually ours. Buddhists and Hindus of all stripes suggest that attachment to the fruits of our labor will bring only disappointment and a terrible sense of unsatisfactoriness.

How does one manage a wild teenager? How do parents keep their children safe and sound during the worst of the hormonal surges of adolescence? Can schools help a student through the worst of it? I really don't know either how we got through it all, or why it was so bad for all of us. In another setting, I would have turned the kids over to a Lakota Sioux medicine man or arranged to have my daughter's bones rattled by a native African healer. Instead, we went the way of other people like us. We enlisted school counselors, male and female psychologists, psychiatrists, and family friends who had passed that way before. In the end, we just held on. And unlike my husband, Giles, I was angry. I was full of rage: angry that the disease had diminished my authority as a parent, angry that Abby could not begin to manage her own life, and angry that she could not seem to figure out how not to get arrested.

Not all patients who come to M. D. Anderson come prepared. Some of them have only a limited understanding of cancer and vague notions about clinical trials, so they remain unsure about their choices. Deb, on the other hand, was as well prepared and as well connected as any patient I had ever met.

She first arrived at the cancer center after having been referred to Dr. Robert Bouquet, the world-famous medical oncologist who discovered CA125, the medical community's best indicator for detecting ovarian cancer. Her surgeon, my chairman, Dr. David Goodman, is world renowned for his work in ovarian cancer at M. D. Anderson, a facility described by *U.S. News & World Report* as one of the best gynecologic cancer centers in the world. Deb's bone marrow transplant was to be directed by Michelle Darling, M.D., a young, very intelligent, and determined woman who essentially ran the bone marrow transplantation program for ovarian cancer patients at M. D. Anderson, and who had earned the respect of everyone in the department. As for me, I was still working my way up the hierarchy, and I wasn't completely sure what my role would be, if any, but I was very fond of Deb, and I wanted to be there for her in any way I could.

I had medical knowledge, of course, but no medical power. From time to time, I would check the hospital computer systems to see if there was anything new on Deb. It's not that her primary physicians didn't want to share the information, but that they didn't know I cared—were unaware of the nature of our evolving relationship. And it's not as if I was sneaking around. I was looking at the results partly because I wanted everything to be okay for her, and partly because *I* needed time to be okay with the results before I faced her.

It was still early in our relationship, however, and I felt as if I was only just beginning to get to know her. During those first few days, as she prepared for the BMT, I barely got a chance to see her. I didn't think I knew her well enough to impose, but one night, shortly after my shift ended, I went off to visit. The lights in her room were turned low, but she was painting, and classical music was playing. Giles was with her. "Well hello, Dr. Lois!" she exclaimed, lighting up. "I was wondering when I was going to see you."

"I didn't want to intrude," I said. "I thought I should give you time to settle in."

"Oh, stop!" she said. "You? Intrude? Never!"

A few days later, I met Abby for the first time. I ran into her outside the hospital entrance, an attractive girl with dyed, jet-black hair and a burning cigarette in her left hand. We exchanged hellos and I told her I was a big fan of her mother's. She smiled politely enough, but without much conviction. In the days ahead, whenever I ran into Abby, I tried to be friendly, I urged her to come to me if she needed to talk. She never did, and she never asked me a direct question, but every time I saw her she smiled and referred to me as "Dr. Lois."

"Abby," I said. "Please stop calling me Dr. Lois. My name is Lois."

"Okay, Dr. Lois," she said. "I'll try."

But I got the impression that I was just another doctor to her—one more person who couldn't tell her anything about the future. She seemed troubled and angry, and she had every right to be. She was just a kid, after all, caught up in a horrible nightmare, and no one had any answers for her.

I have for some time now wanted to write about this period in our lives and our experience in the world of elite secondary education. It might serve as a form of catharsis to describe the frustration and despair I experienced at the hands of these private institutions and the administrators, counselors, and psychologists that run them.

It started during Abby's first year at the Gibson School, 1999–2000, when I fell out of the Remission Society, and continued well into her second year. Gibson made our difficult lives even more difficult. While it was clear we were not in a position to endow a building or a lectureship, we paid our bills on time, and I volunteered to help students working on projects involving Buddhism and Hindu tradition.

And then there was Abby. A drama queen by nature, she had starred in the school production of Sister Mary Ignatius Explains It All to You. Written by a very angry and very well educated ex-Catholic, the play uses Catholic ideology to justify the sadistic behavior of Sister Mary, which culminates with Sister Mary's murder of two of her former students. Was the Gibson administration afraid that life would imitate art? Sister Mary was clearly mad. Did this mean that Abby was, too? After all, she was extraordinarily convincing, lecturing the audience on the differences between venal and moral sins and on the placement, in limbo, of dead babies who had not had the benefit of baptism.

In the life of the school, Abby became the site where many Gibson students could live out their own fears about abandonment and the death of a beloved parent. Abby's psychological drama, including her exclamation that she would kill herself if her mother died, became the occasion for the Gibson administration to further limit her movements at the school. In a conversation with the school's headmaster, I pointed out that even my doctors didn't think I would die before the end of the school year, and in fact, Abby's *exclamation, to use the Latin, was expressed in the subjunctive. It was a conditional phrase: If this happens, then I will do this—"I will kill myself." It was not declarative, nor was it vocative.*

In truth, of course, my disease and Abby's behavior had become just too much for the school to manage. This was a place of pastoral dreams. Illness was an uninvited guest. Other students with sick parents had been offered the opportunity to leave school and return home.

We survived Gibson, but I still bear the administration a grudge and wish a pox on their houses. I remember too well the late-night phone calls from administrators who never tired of assuring me that Abby had a good deal of support on campus. On the heels of one such call, literally an hour later, Abby was placed on medical leave from the school. It clearly did not occur to them that I myself was on medical leave and that I was in no shape to manage a distraught teenager at home. My husband, Giles, was teaching some twenty-five miles away, and the kid did not drive.

After an appeal to the headmaster, Abby was allowed to attend classes but was denied routine privileges, marking her with the stigma of ostracism, one of the poisons most potent to adolescents. Despite the adults' rhetoric and the sheer beauty of the school's grounds, it was a cruel and punishing place. Even in my diminished state I did what I could to make the lives of Gibson teachers and Gibson parents uncomfortable. I wrote repeatedly to the Gibson administrators who were responsible for students' health and welfare, and finally, I wrote to the mother of one of Abby's peers who had gone directly to the headmaster to demand that Abigail Gunn be expelled from Gibson School. Alas, it was only a letter-writing campaign. Nevertheless, on Abby's last day at Gibson, the headmaster did say to her that he wished they "had done it better."

Why did my kids' behavior make me so angry? As with most people, rage is born of a kind of grief. My own childhood was filled with family illness and terrible trouble. Infant death, my mother's decline into alcoholism, blindness for my father at sixty. At about the same time, my then seventeen-year-old brother began a siege with ulcerative colitis that left him, a year later, with a colostomy and some degree of madness. Dr. Sun argues that adversity and human difficulties make for a more substantive person. This may be true, but most of us would say that we could do without either. When I behaved badly, I did it after I was over eighteen years of age.

Having lived a life too much in service of the kids, I was outraged that illness now wanted the rest of the life that was left to me. I wanted what was left of my life. I had had enough of their lives. It is the standard despairing mother's response: "Look what I gave up for you and this is how you treat me!" I wanted them to stand with me in this fight against the forces of darkness, but they had their own demons to fight.

Was it simply rage born of grief that convulsed our family? Abby became a problem that competed with cancer. Incidences of stealing and cutting were part of the fabric of our lives, along with chemotherapy, birthday parties, and walks with the dogs.

Hanging over everything, of course, was the cancer—adding to my sadness and my anger. As I discovered in due course, patients can sometimes blame the messenger in cancer care. This has *always struck me as a foolish way to proceed. The messenger in cancer care is often also the surgeon or the medical oncologist who will define the strategy for treatment. Entering the Kingdom of the Ill and coming to terms with a cancer diagnosis is difficult, but it is important to remember that while these physicians and nurses will be part of your world for the remainder of your life, they didn't give you the disease. The cancer began somewhere else. The human difficulty of coming to accept a life one didn't choose for oneself, and the requirement that one behave in a civil and humane manner, can be very trying. I have seen and participated in all sorts of strange and finally useless responses to this human dilemma.*

I also went, very briefly and against my better judgment, to a support group for women with cancer. I heard a lovely young mother, recently diagnosed with breast cancer, shout to the women who would listen—a group of about twelve—that her surgeon had done her terrible harm, and that she and her husband and their two-year-old daughter were about to leave for Mexico, where they could secure real care, including some form of coffee enemas and laetrile (an apricot pit extract). Her husband, a scientist of sorts, had explained to her, and then she to us, just how this drug combination would work. This support group was convened by the American Cancer Center and chaired by a licensed social worker.

Out of curiosity, and with a degree of incredulity, I went back for one more meeting, mostly to ask why no one had tried to stop this clearly agitated woman from turning away from standard treatment. Everyone at the meeting had simply smiled and nodded, apparently having no opinion on the matter. Then the social worker explained that her work—and, really, the work of the oncologic team—was to present the options to the patient and to let the patient and her family decide how to proceed. I then asked, "What if anger and rage born of grief cloud a patient's mind, making clear thinking impossible?"

"That is not our problem," the social worker told me.

Not long after, I happened to overhear a conversation between two gynecologic oncologists, and I realized that my own mind had become somewhat cloudy. With some irony, one physician said to the other that 90 percent of his ovarian cancer patients thought they were among the 10 percent who would survive the disease.

I was clearly part of that 90 percent. I had to be. I refused to accept the possibility that I might be dying.

4

THE GREAT EQUALIZER

I didn't have a teenage daughter in trouble with the law, but it certainly didn't feel like things at my home were much better.

By now, Ross and I had already given up on even trying to share a quick meal together—had practically given up talking, to be honest—and it was becoming increasingly clear to both of us that we were in serious trouble. Sometimes, briefly, our schedules would overlap, and I'd return home to find him parked in front of the TV, flipping channels, too exhausted to do much more than greet me from afar. It was at times like those that I despaired. *We are living separate lives,* I would think. *There is no hope for us. And worse, we don't seem to care.*

Before long, we were strangers who just happened to be living under the same roof, and the only thing we had in common was the beautiful daughter we'd brought into the world.

Still, there were moments when the distance and the indifference really got to me, and I would engage him, knowing it would turn into an argument, but still feeling somehow that that connection was better than bland indifference. At times like those, we would find ourselves exorcising our frustrations by yelling at each other.

"You could stand up and say hello when I walk into the house!"

"I'm tired, too! I just finished a twelve-hour shift!"

Jessica hated the yelling as much as we did, and she often complained of tummyaches to get us to stop. But even when we weren't yelling, we were communicating very badly. I remember telling Jessica to brush her teeth one night—a rare night when the three of us were home together, in body, if not in spirit—and she refused. I turned to Ross and said, "Help me out here, would you?" And he said snidely, "I don't really think kids need to brush their teeth twice a day." I was shocked. "I can't believe you just said that," I told him. I couldn't believe he would put his need to score a point in an argument against me over doing what was best for Jessie. "Is this what it has come to? Is this how far gone we are?"

Don't get me wrong: Ross was a terrific guy, but he wasn't the guy for me—and I wasn't the girl for him. When we were in medical school, we got married without really thinking about it. We went to classes, studied hard, worked, and seldom focused on the deeper issues—the issues that really mattered. Now that we had demanding jobs, and a child, we focused on those issues even less. That's how it felt to me, anyway. Instead of helping each other become the best possible versions of ourselves, we were criticizing and attacking each other for all the ways we were disappointed in where we found ourselves.

One night, I found Deb alone in her room, and she told me about the unhappy experience with that support group in Santa Barbara. "It was terrible," she said. "Not only did they make no sense, but I was forced to identify with women who are ill. I don't want to identify with the ill. I want to identify with the well."

It was tough to argue with that, and tough to know what to say. If you don't believe you're going to make it, why bother struggling?

Managing one's interior life after a cancer diagnosis is a difficult business, and one needs all the help pharmacological, practical, spiritual, social—of which one can avail oneself. Most religious traditions tell us that it is fear that really ruins a life. We are all fearful and weak creatures, so says Christianity's St. Augustine. Desire for more leads to our terror of having less, say the Buddhists, and—for the Jews—fear of the Lord is a good thing. It stands before, and diminishes, smaller human fears about death, loss, and betrayal. Everyone in cancer care is afraid. For some it is the first real encounter with the imminent prospect of dying, and often, the proposed treatment—at least in some ways—sounds as if it had been devised by one of Satan's minions on the fourth level of hell. For the layperson, let me just say that chemotherapy and radiation are both a form of cooking, and that the body heats up accordingly.

A number of cancer survivors have written narratives of their experience when having a bone marrow transplant—BMT to the initiated. Generally speaking, this is your last best hope. It is difficult even now to write with any clarity about the experience. It is a carefully orchestrated drama, a drama that involves hospitalizations followed by days of outpatient care, which are then again followed by another hospitalization and, if all goes well, a final medical release.

In nonmedical terms, the theory behind a BMT is quite simple. One is given so much chemotherapy that one dies—but in the case of the BMT, life is maintained by other means. These other means involve the use of antibiotics, blood or platelet transfusions, hydration, and God knows what else. The argument is simple: If the patient dies, then perhaps the cancer will die with her.

There are a variety of ways to do a BMT with high-dose chemotherapy. My treatment involved two rounds of chemo. The first round required a three-day, round-the-clock infusion. The second round, given several weeks later, after millions of little Deb stem cells had been collected, involved a five-day course of chemo, given each morning. After a day off, I was then infused with a bag of little Deb stem cells. I then descended into what the Muslims would call "occultation," then waited for the little Deb stem cells to find their way into my bones and jump-start the life process. This waiting can last from eight days to two weeks.

BMT began my friendship with Dr. Michelle Darling, who orchestrated my procedure. I spoke with her over the telephone immediately after I learned of this recurrence. I could not place her accent; while her English was flawless, it was not her first language. As I learned later, when I met Dr. Darling for the first time, she is Canadian from Montreal and her first language is French. In addition to English, I believe she also speaks Italian. She is a consummate artist who works in oils and on really big canvases. She is a reader and a thinker and a master builder, as students of gematria would put it, and Dr. Bouquet describes her as the very best transplanter working in the field today. And while she is in her midthirties, she looks about twelve. I have no idea how this informs her working life with colleagues and patients, but at least in me it invokes a sense of my own adolescence and a sense of the maternal. She needs none of this, of course, yet my life, quite apart from the ovarian cancer problem, is better for having had her in it. Quite apart from her intrinsic character—a personality that possesses a "whim of iron," to quote an old friend—she is thoughtful beyond measure and has enabled me to move my own thinking and devotion to art to new areas.

As my life of mobility declines, my time devoted to art enlarges, and it is to Dr. Darling that I am most grateful for the encouragement and the conversation that has provided me with a measure of courage, and finally humor, to paint canvases as well as blocks of wood, to use the scissors and a stapler, and, finally, to conceive of a "golem series"—a series that draws on my limited knowledge of Jewish Kabbalah and my imaginative life of the golem redux.

Professor Temple Grandin has argued for the humane treat-

ment of cattle as they are readied for slaughter. She writes about getting the cattle ready and relaxed for death by putting them into a "squeeze chute," which administers pressure that calms the cattle as they walk up the passageway toward the processing area. Signing up for a BMT is a little like deciding to enter the chute. A series of releases must be signed, all of which end with the tagline "May result in. . . . " It is, using Arnold van Gennup's categories, "a rite of passage." The BMT really can change your life. In some cancer cases, but not in all, the BMT can cure you.

The BMT drama is difficult and, from what I have learned, is more difficult for some than for others. One of my dearest nurses, Jackie, told me of a case she encountered when she had just joined the staff of the BMT service. A young man, full of life, had been diagnosed with a form of lymphoma that required a BMT. It meant that this vital and athletic fellow would be sequestered in a room and visited only by people in masks for about four weeks. Near the end of his trial, so Jackie related the story to me, he informed her that he had had enough and that he had to get out. Before she could reply, he had ripped the various needles and tubing from his arms and chest and run out of the room to the hospital elevator. Blood was abundant and the level of alarm palpable. He was eventually returned to his room and was supplied with a stationary bicycle. The stationary bicycle became standard equipment for the young and athletic.

I did no such thing. On a good day I would play my violin. On a not-so-good day I would watch a video of a performance of State Street Ballet or paint a picture. In the morning, the Texas sun was luminous, giving the room the quality of a Monet painting. Of course, the room also had a television set. All hospital rooms by definition have a television set: It is part of the room's equipment. For the most part, television is a sick person's version of sociability. I could not watch television while I was undergoing the BMT. I couldn't tolerate the uncertainty of television commercials or any kind of programming. There was too much anxiety involved in it for me. I did not know what was going to happen next, either on the screen or in my life. I had so little control over the life that was before me that the uncertainty of television was simply too much to bear. I wanted no surprises in a life that had proved to be too full of them.

What one learned came from one's blood counts. Every morning at about 5:00 A.M. a masked phlebotomist, usually a lovely and congenial woman, would come into my room and extract some blood from the catheter in my chest. Later in the day, the flock of physicians, all in white coats, would come in and report the result. For the most part, it was a ritualized visit. I wanted to look my best—lipstick and earrings—but they came and went with a swoosh. The team involved pharmacists as well as physicians and medical fellows, both male and female. I knew only the leader of the team.

Hospitalized twice during this BMT drama, I had two different team leaders and two very different experiences. On the first I remain very keen. Dr. Donte was originally from South America. A wonderfully engaging human being, Dr. Donte was recently married and was expecting his first child. Both my husband and I had read Machado de Assis's The Posthumous Memoirs of Bras Cubas. It is the equivalent in his home country of The Scarlet

Letter, *the book by Nathaniel Hawthorne to which Americans attach so much pride and affection. All children in Brazil read this "autobiography," written, as the author tells us, after his death. Both Giles and I realized that Dr. Donte did not often have the opportunity to discuss his country's literature with his patients or even his colleagues at the hospital. Our conversations moved from literature to architecture, then to music and to art. It was delightful to have him as my physician while I was "in house." Often his colleagues would leave us to continue our discussion after we had moved away from medical matters.*

During my second stay in the hospital, I had a much less talkative physician who led the BMT team on morning rounds. Dr. Kella was reserved in the way that Dr. Donte was expansive. He had a good deal to do each morning and did not want to waste time engaging patients in nonmedical chatter. Too, given my general condition during the transplant, I was in good shape—at least compared with some of the other patients. Dr. Kella was responsible for the infusion of the millions of little Deb stem cells that presumably would bring me back to life, a second birthday of sorts, a resurrection if you will, complete with Mylar balloons and a crowd. The infusion takes only a few minutes, and I celebrated, as many patients do, by throwing up.

As Deb clearly saw, too, there is a kind of strangeness in cancer care and in cancer centers. The world is a different place. All bets are off, one might say; the focus is on living. The rest doesn't matter as much, at least not to most patients.

I think the constant exposure to this type of care changes caregivers, whether they know it or not, and I was no exception. I saw myself literally becoming a different person. I wanted to break out of the narrow circle that defined my life, into this larger world—strange as it was.

I remember getting into the elevator one day, and a nurse hopped on behind me, a man close on her heels. The man greeted the nurse with some jollity. As the elevator climbed, he made light conversation, and she responded in a friendly manner. Then the elevator stopped and the door opened, and they got off, and I heard the nurse asking about his wife. As the doors closed, he said, "I am hoping God takes her today. I can't stand to see her suffer anymore." The doors closed, and I was alone in the elevator. I then thought, as Deb had said many times: *Lois, you're not in Kansas anymore.*

Truly, the world of the hospital is a strange place. Other people are worried about Iraq, or about terrorism, or about their retirement fund, or about global warming, but at M. D. Anderson most people are literally hanging on for dear life. The others—the families of the patients—are in a strange world of their own. Every time I ran into Giles, for example, he was full of questions. How was the treatment going? What could he expect? Where could he look for the most current research? Was there anything promising on the horizon? His main concern, his *only* concern, really, was how to save his wife.

During my fellowship, I saw all kinds of husbands. Some had bailed out long before I even met the patient. These husbands may have divorced their wives out of fear, lack of education, absent compassion, or, simply, just a selfish wish for an easier life—a healthier, easier *wife*.

Sometimes I met men who attempted to cage and tame their anxieties by bringing such familiar tools as a lined notebook and pencil to each doctor's visit. I thought of these husbands as "The Engineers." They always took detailed notes, asked many questions, and repeated my words to make themselves feel as if they had at least *some* control. They were trying to fix the situation for their wives in the best way they knew how. Other husbands, "The Worriers," sat in the room and said nothing—overwhelmed, possibly, by their own mortality—and became meek and childlike. Then there were those who asked more questions than the patient asked, and kept asking them, as if maybe the answer would change and everything would turn out as they'd hoped.

Deb's husband, Giles, seemed to fall somewhere between the engineer and the worrier. He is an accomplished author of many books on things as various as cultural theory and criticism, American literature, philosophy, religion, and, most recently, global studies—books that I have been embarrassed to tell him I could not easily follow. Although initially intimidating to me—the stature, the bass voice, the impressive academic credentials—I soon came to see him in a completely different light, as a good man and a wonderfully supportive husband. He was at Deb's side every step of the way, and he was intimately involved in all decisions related to her treatment. He put his career on hold in order to care for his family, and I never heard him utter a single word of complaint. His wife needed him and he was going to be there for her. It didn't get any simpler than that.

As you might imagine, cancer is not just the patient's disease, but a family illness. Everyone in a family will be affected, and everyone will experience the cancer in his or her own way. They are victims, too. Some families will be pulled apart by the experience, others will find ways to live full lives despite the cancer, and others still—the majority, perhaps—will fall squarely in the middle. There are victims in every battle, but not every battle produces heroes and not every battle exposes cowards. We are all just people here, trying to make sense of this business of living.

Giles was a special case. He seemed to have a knack for reading his wife's needs. He was courageous one moment, tearful the next, and always uncritically attentive to Deb.

When the family arrived in Houston to prepare for the BMT, Deb was angry about both the cancer and the troubles with Abby. "I'm the one that's sick, and I have to deal with her shit," she told me.

"It's hard for her, too," I said. "To see you sick. It's very frightening."

"I know, I know. When you're a teenager, the world is supposed to revolve around you. But instead the world revolves around your mother and her cancer."

"Have you talked to her about it?"

"I've tried, but what am I supposed to tell her? 'Don't worry, Abby! Everything's going to be just fine!'? It's not going to be just fine. It's not going to be fine at all."

Despite everything, Deb was trying very hard to be a good mother and a good wife. She once told me that she didn't like having Giles in the room when her doctors came to her with updates on her condition, because then she'd have to worry about his reaction. "I feel like I should process the information first, so that we don't both get upset at the same time," she explained. "I guess it's a form of managing family anxiety."

Family anxiety—now that was a topic I knew a little something about, if for completely different reasons. By this point, it was clear that Ross and I were headed for divorce. I had been to see a therapist, and I bought books on marriage and how to make it work, but none of it helped—we were beyond help. At one point, Ross came with me to see the therapist, but even the therapist could see that it was over. We talked about the lack of intimacy, and about the things we liked and disliked in each other, and it soon became apparent that there wasn't much of a marriage left to save. "You seem to have lost your way," the therapist told us. I thought that was the understatement of the year. I did not feel connected to my husband anymore, on any level.

At work I tried to keep my feelings to myself, but as my shift drew to a close I allowed myself the luxury of thinking about my daughter, and I would be filled with joy at the prospect of seeing her. Inevitably, however, just as I was about to walk out the door, one of my superiors would say, "Lois, there's one more thing you need to do before you leave." I would do it, and I usually held myself together, but on my way home I often fell apart—and then I'd feel guilty about falling apart. *These women are sick,* I'd think. *What's your excuse?*

One night, Ross and I were arguing, *again*, as Jessie played nearby. As our voices reached a fever pitch, she looked up at us and said, "My tummy hurts." Her little face was twisted.

I felt like I'd been stabbed in the heart. I looked at Ross. At that moment, we both realized that we couldn't keep doing this—that even Jessie was unhappy.

"Are you miserable?" he asked.

"Yes," I said. It was surprisingly easy to admit. "Aren't you?"

He took a moment. "I've been looking around at apartments," he said quietly.

Oddly, I was relieved.

My parents weren't, though. "It's a marriage," my mother said. "You make it work."

I spoke to my sister, Karen, from time to time, looking for a little support, but she was in a solid marriage and was caring for two kids, and I always felt—right or wrong—that my unhappiness was hard for her to understand.

I would remind myself that I wasn't unique. I knew six people who were married while still in med school, and five of them were already divorced. Still, I would wonder. Why couldn't we have been the ones to make it work?

There was a six-month period when I was so scattered that I got into three minor fender-benders. One of my friends sent me flowers, as a joke. On the card, she had written: "Thanks from all the autobody-repair shops in Pearland, Texas!"

I finally got back into jogging, thinking it might help. Every morning at the crack of dawn I'd run with a girlfriend from the hospital, and I would talk about my crumbling marriage for the duration of the run. I'm sure it was hard on her, but for me it was great therapy.

Talking to Deb also proved very therapeutic. Often I would be trying to discuss something about her medical regimen, but then she'd turn the conversation around. She had a knack for that. "So how's Jess? What's going on with Ross? Did he find an apartment yet?"

"Why are we talking about my trivial little problems?" I said. "I'm here to talk about you."

"Oh, I'm fine—given the circumstances," she replied. "You're a much more interesting person. I'm an academic; you're curing cancer. You're saving the lives of women."

"Working on it," I said.

"So, come on—what's happening at home?"

"Ross isn't a bad guy," I said. "We just, you know—we never really got beyond the surface stuff. He's a great father, though. I'll give him that much."

"You have to get beyond the 'surface stuff,'" she said. "A marriage, like a close friendship, is an ongoing conversation. If you lose interest in the person, if you no longer have anything to say to each other, it's over."

Strangely, Deb made me realize that one doesn't get anywhere by trying to measure the seriousness of a problem or by comparing it to other problems. I sat with dying people every day, and I would see the photographs by their hospital beds—of family, of friends, of themselves in better days, with big smiles and full heads of hair—and I would think, *My life is easy. What am I complaining about?* But on my way home I'd get a flat tire, or a ticket for not coming to a complete stop at the corner, and I'd become so upset that I was actually ashamed of my response. And before long I began to see that the daily problems, big and small, were less important than *how* I responded to them, and I began to get a little better at handling my daily frustrations. I'm not there yet, but I'm still working on it, and I still have a long way to go.

Finally, the big day came. "Ross is moving out," I told Deb.

"Oh, Lois," she said, and she sighed deeply.

"It's hard," I admitted.

"Listen to me," she said. "I am full of advice, and much of it is wrong, but I'm unquestionably on your side. This is an ending, but it is not *the* end, and you are going to continue."

I felt connected to Deb in ways I didn't fully understand. I felt as if she had come into my life for a reason. I felt that she was opening doors for me, doors I hadn't even known existed.

After the BMT, when she had regained some of her strength, she again moved into Rotary House, where she turned the room she and Giles shared into an apartment. She would play classical music and paint, experimenting with folk art, especially with the golems she had talked about. These were manlike creatures from Jewish folklore, popularized in certain Kabbalistic stories.

Every time I visited Deb, she would ask about my life at home. She had a gift for pulling things out of me that I wouldn't share with anyone else, not even my devoted jogging partner.

"Ross doesn't want to hire a lawyer," I told Deb. "He said he knows I'll be fair."

"So you see?" she said. "He does know a *little* about you."

When the time came to file for the actual divorce, Ross gave me a notarized letter and asked me to handle it. We later had to attend a class on divorce etiquette, as mandated by Texas law, and we went separately. I listened to what I already knew: *Don't fight in front of your kids. Never say anything bad about your ex in front of the kids. Remember that you are going to be the child's parents for the rest of your lives.* I liked hearing it anyway. A little reinforcement goes a long way.

I was still a mess, of course. I was still jogging with my friend several mornings a week, swatting the Texas-sized mosquitoes every step of the way, and still feeling actively sorry for myself.

"I am such a failure," I told Deb.

"I'm not even going to honor that with a response," Deb said, laughing.

One day I was leafing through the local paper and saw an ad for salsa classes in my neighborhood. I thought it might be a good way to take my mind off my troubles—Deb had talked often about the therapeutic effects of dancing—so I signed up. It worked. When I was dancing, I forgot everything else. When I was dancing, I felt free. I didn't miss a class.

A few weeks later, my family came to visit—a postdivorce support mission, I guess. My sister, Karen, also came, with her two kids. One evening we went for a walk around a nearby lake.

As Jessie talked and played with her cousins, I dropped back to talk to my sister. "Can you believe it?" I said wryly. "I'm a single mom, stuck in Pearland, Texas. How the hell did this happen?"

At least we were able to laugh about it.

I introduced my parents to Deb during this visit. We met at the Empire Café, a Houston coffee shop, and they were both very taken with her, but I could see that my father was uncomfortable with the whole idea of illness and death. Deb looked pretty good, all things considered—the lipstick, the earrings—but she was definitely, as she put it, in the Kingdom of the Ill. My mother was quite impressed. "She's very classy," she said.

"Yes," I said. "And she's like a magnet. She looks at you and you feel yourself being drawn to her, almost encompassed by her."

At one point, my mother decided she felt comfortable enough around Deb to complain about me. "Lois's e-mails are very short," she said. "All I get is a sentence or two. And usually she doesn't even put my name on top."

Deb immediately came to my defense, bless her heart. "Don't take it personally," she said. "Your daughter is a Healer in a Hurry."

Before my parents left, my father took me aside and said, "Whatever you need, you know we're here for you."

"Thank you," I said.

In the weeks that followed, I stole away to visit Deb whenever possible. There were bad days, when she felt she was living on borrowed time, and there were days when she felt she had finally beaten this thing. "You know, Lois, I don't want to die, but I don't want to hang on when there's no reason left to hang on," she said. "Do you understand what I'm saying?"

"I do."

"When the time comes to let go, *if* the time comes to let go, I hope I have the courage to do so. And if I don't, I hope you're there to set me straight."

"It's a little early to be making promises," I said, and she laughed her big laugh.

During this period I got to know both Giles and Abby a little better. Abby was still struggling, understandably, with the fact that her mother had a fatal illness, and still recovering from her experiences with the private school back home. But now that she was in Houston with her family, where they could keep an eye on her, keep her close and safe, she seemed to be adapting fairly well. She even seemed to be enjoying the large, multiracial school to which she'd transferred, the cultural shock notwithstanding.

Lamar Public High School had thirty-five hundred kids, a third white, a third African American, and a third Latino. I was there for Abby, trying to be a parent, but I was not always fully present, so the full weight of helping her cope fell largely to Giles.

Teenagers, even without a really sick parent, can have a difficult time of it. Most good children's literature begins with the death
of a parent. Roald Dahl makes it a prerequisite to the start of every
story. Dickens's protagonists often have to deal with the aftereffects
of losing a mother. David Copperfield and Oliver Twist are the
obvious examples. However, there is not too much written on how
to live during what the young person imagines to be the period of
parental decline—the dress rehearsal for dying.

It also runs counter to expectations. The teenager is preparing him or herself to leave home, to become independent, and to
make a life. The teenager is supposed to leave, not the parent.
Too, in the world of cancer care, there is so much to do. A parent
who had been doting and devoted is transformed into a patient
whose main interest is the condition of the self. I remember a
young girl, Shirley, about fourteen, who befriended Abby immediately after we arrived at M. D. Anderson for my bone marrow
transplantation. I expected to be sequestered in the hospital, on
and off, for three months, and none of us were looking forward
to it.

Shirley's mother was already in "the chute," as they say, and
Shirley had come from Florida to see her. A short time later
her mother passed away. When Shirley stopped by to tell me that
her mother had died, a strange smile crossed her face. There was
no sense that this smile had any connection to her feelings for her
mother. It reflected instead the sense of an ending. The drama was
over. Shirley didn't have to be anxious or wait anymore. It was
finished. And I understood it. Certainly my daughter and son felt
this way, too. How long can this go on?

Abby finished the first semester of her sophomore year at Lamar High School, and she had a fairly interesting life there. She was cast as Abigail Brewster in Joseph Kesselring's wonderfully funny play Arsenic and Old Lace.

Chubby, wearing old-lady shoes and a wig with a snood, re-imagining herself as an eccentric but well-heeled member of the Daughters of the American Revolution, Abby and her friend Claire, who played the other sister, carried the show. Murdering old men at will with the help of their nephew, who thought of himself as President Theodore Roosevelt, they buried the yellow fever victims who were helping to build the Panama Canal in the basement. They were incredible. I will never know how she managed this theatrical feat while she was sleeping through many of her classes, but she did.

While I was in the hospital, or plugged into some hydrating source at the Rotary House, Giles did his best to keep an eye on her, but she seldom turned in before three or four in the morning, and he was always exhausted. It goes without saying that getting her to school in the morning was quite difficult.

It was also a hard time for our son, Adam, who was back in California, trying to figure out how to get on with his life, and what, exactly, that meant. *Illness is genuinely crazy-making.*

One of the psychologists at M. D. Anderson explained that children have to learn how "to keep themselves safe," and that every child is different. At the end of the day, she said, it is not important how they manage it, but that they manage it successfully.

I enjoy the company of my children, and I especially enjoy their laughter. I share their troubles and give advice when asked. I even give them advice when they don't ask, but I don't expect that they will take it. And apart from Giles, there is no one else's company I enjoy as much as theirs.

I am also very much enjoying Dr Lois, the two of us still dancing our way around each other. How does one describe friendship between two women, one thirteen years older than the other? One is a physician of extraordinary skill, the other an antiquarian of sorts—with a little bit of knowledge about a good many things. According to the New York Review of Books, Nancy Mitford described her friend Mrs. Esther Murphy Arthur as "a large sandy person like a bedroom cupboard packed full of information, much of it useless, all of it accurate." I am neither large nor sandy, but I do possess a great deal of accurate information, and I use it freely in my teaching and in my conversations. I am also curious, and I was and remain curious about Dr. Lois's views of the world.

I sometimes imagine that if I am quiet enough and concentrate, I can see Dr. Lois think. I can feel the connections she is making between this and that. What makes her so interesting is perhaps the very thing that makes me useless. I have lived on the margins. I am a commentator. If I go into class and tell my students that the French Revolution started in 1889, I can go in the next day and tell them I was wrong, off by a hundred years. Dr. Lois and the community of physicians do not have this luxury, nor do they live with this ease of forgiveness. We all make mistakes, physicians and teachers alike, yet for Dr. Lois the consequences are apparent, sometimes immediate, and in terrible cases, deadly. Does it help that Dr. Lois is helping her patient fight what is surely death itself? I would think it does, but the immediacy of suffering is real, no matter the inevitable outcome.

I could not do cancer work. I could not be a physician, and I am grateful to the fates that other people can find the grit and the courage to do it instead.

Deb was right in saying that friendship, like marriage, was an ongoing conversation. I had never had a friendship quite like this one, and I valued it immensely. I also think it was making me a better doctor. I was able to see, firsthand, what Deb and her family were going through—was able to share in the emotional toll. If I'd had any reservations, ethical or emotional, about getting too close to patients, they were gone. Deb was taking me farther inside the worries, fears, and hopes of all my patients, and that couldn't possibly be a bad thing.

I remember another patient—another of my Amazing Women—who came in around that time. She had a huge tumor in her belly, a tumor so large and pronounced that I could feel it through her skin. She was unable to eat, and so frail that a strong gust of wind could have blown her over. I told her that we would have to start with chemotherapy, and I explained the process as succinctly as possible: Chemo kills quickly growing cells, the cancer cells. These cells grow quickly because they have lost their "off" switch. But in the process of killing them, some normal cells die also—blood cells, platelets, white cells, hair cells, etc.—so a healthy part of the patient is sacrificed to kill the intruders. The problem arises when we don't kill all the bad cells, however, because those will continue to grow, and the cancer will recur. That is why we need to be aggressive.

"Do you understand what I'm telling you?" I asked her.

"I think so," she said.

"After the chemo, we can operate and see what else we can do for you. Okay?"

"I'm going to rely on God to give me strength," she said.

"That's good," I said. "I need you to be strong."

"I will, Dr. Lois, but please don't go away. Jesus will be here, but I'm going to need you, too."

How could I begrudge her that need for closeness? And really, what was wrong with it? I was beginning to see it as my duty. Other doctors might disagree, particularly those who focus so intently on the illness that they don't even see the patient, but I wanted to be as present as I possibly could, and I had chosen a field that allowed me to do so.

Let me explain: The role of the gynecologic oncologist is very different from that of the medical oncologist or the surgical oncologist, primarily because we make both the surgical and medical treatment decisions. The gynecologic oncologist is the physician of reference for the entire course of the patient's illness. As a result, he or she really has an opportunity to get to know his patients, and to connect with them as human beings.

Deb had an arrangement that was considerably different from that of the average patient. She had two medical oncologists, one in Santa Barbara and one in Houston, as well as her gynecologic surgical oncologist, and, more recently, her

BMT specialist (not to mention a radiation oncologist). Deb's care was multidisciplinary, but she was so charismatic that she forged unusual friendships with almost all of her physicians. Though their days were overbooked already, most of them made time for her.

Deb and I often talked about the relationship between patients and doctors, about communication in general, and specifically about the BMT experience. The bone marrow transplantation service at M. D. Anderson runs patient care slightly differently from its other surgical services. Very often, medical services work in shifts, focusing at times on patient care and resident teaching, and at other times on research and paper writing. Although this may be acceptable for some patients, whose general obstetrician-gynecologist may or may not be generally readily available, it is an entirely different experience for the cancer patient—a patient who is dying and is struggling to understand why. Treating a pregnant woman who is awaiting the birth of her child with great hope and a sense of awe is one thing; treating a dying patient who is preparing to step into the Great Unknown is quite another.

Deb found that the on-and-off service technique of the bone marrow transplantation service was less than desirable for a patient who had relocated her family. She was worried about her chances of survival, and she often felt nauseated and weak. Throughout, however, she remained adamant about being seen as a real person, not as a sick patient.

"My doctor should know who I am," she told me more

than once, and I will never forget the power of that statement. *My doctor should know who I am.* "There's much more to lose than a medical life," she explained. "There's one's imaginative life, one's artistic life, one's intellectual life. This is what's at stake, and to recognize it is the beginning of spirituality in medicine."

My relationship with Deb taught me that I should always fight for closeness. I do not expect to have equally intense relationships with all of my patients, but it is critical for me to get to know them as individuals. Unfortunately, this is not part of our training. There is no time for it.

During our first year as gynecologic fellows, we spend two years in the laboratory learning basic science techniques. Some of us have some previous knowledge of these techniques; some of us have none. It is quite a difficult process, moving from a completed residency program in obstetrics and gynecology, where one has mastered the field of delivering babies, to essentially restarting at the bottom of the totem pole in the remotely related subject of cancer, death, and the dying.

Obstetric and gynecology residents usually get very little training in cancer care. Depending on the residency program, most residents in this field approach the cancer elective as one in which they don't really need to know anything. The only emotion it really promotes is distant sympathy, or, worse, a degree of apathy.

Now that I train residents, I usually hand them a list of ten reasons to be enthusiastic about oncology, hoping that one of them will sink in. My number one reason: "The patients are all your mothers, sisters, or possibly you." Farther down the list of reasons is one that is a tad self-serving: "Being enthusiastic will make your attending physician [me] happy."

There are of course patients who are difficult and even unpleasant, and then it's more of a struggle to be compassionate. But as I tell my residents, "They are the ones who are dying. Not you. You have to get beyond it. Just do everything you can, then go back and do it a little better."

Of course, none of us are perfect. I tend to be impatient, and from time to time I've been known to lose my temper with trainees. I've also been told, by more than one superior, that I have the tenacity of a pit bull. In the context of that discussion, I believe this was a compliment, but that doesn't make it any easier on my trainees (I know for a fact that some have referred to me, behind my back, as Dr. *Rambo*-detta. I take that as a compliment, too). I'm serious about medicine, but I am not completely without humor. Often in the middle of a surgery, I've been known to say, "If you cut that, I am going to have to kill you." It works every time. The trainee takes a deep breath, considers his or her potential mistake, and survives—as does the patient.

Still, patience is not my strong suit, and I am not always generous with my trainees, and on more than one occasion I've thought about private practice. But I can't do it. I will remain in an academic setting because I would like to continue to participate in the search for a potential cancer cure.

As for the patients, I never forget—and I never let my trainees forget—that they are *my* patients. These women have entrusted me to take them safely through the operation and recovery, and if I'm going to get help from a resident or fellow, as I know I must, I will be watching them like a hawk.

One of my early teachers used to say, "To do a good job you have to always check what you did. Then check again. And when you're sure you got it right, check one more time." That's the level of commitment I expect from my students, and I don't think I need to apologize for it. Unfortunately, many of them are just there to get through gynecologic oncology. This is a depressing field to most of them, and they just want to put it behind them and plunge into the happy business of delivering babies.

Not long ago, I wrote a letter to a friend who was having second thoughts about going into the field. I told her about one of my earliest mentors, Dr. Bunton, a rough-on-the-outside but deeply empathic man, and about the powerful effect he had on me and my fellow trainees: "It is not necessarily that we wanted to please him, but that we wanted to *be* like him. He gained our respect because of his behavior, clinical skills, and the personal thought he devoted to his patients' care, and also for the love he had for his family. That is what we wanted. Even when we felt we wanted to be home with our families, through him we learned that there would be plenty of time for that, too."

Shortly after receiving my letter, my friend started her fellowship in gynecologic oncology. Things didn't turn out as either of us had hoped. She found herself overwhelmingly depressed by the situations she was forced to confront on a daily basis, and she went into a different field. If she had hung in there, she might have learned that it is okay to have these feelings. I have them every day: *I like this patient, and the odds are I'm going to lose her, and I know what it means to her and her family, and it's going to hurt.*

You hang on. You talk to them. And you listen—above all, you listen. And then one day, when all hope is gone, you have to have The Talk. You need to tell them that you can keep trying to extend their life, but that it's not going to be much of a life. You need to tell them to start thinking about the *quality* of life that's left to them, not the quantity.

Unfortunately, some doctors are just not very good at this conversation. It's hard, it's painful, it often feels like an admission of defeat, and—more than anything else—it forces the doctors to deal with their *own* mortality. They want to stay in "Kansas." They may be good doctors, but their inability to have these types of conversations is not good for them, and not good for their patients.

Often, I tell my students, "You know you're getting close to needing to discuss end-of-life decisions when you reach a patient's door and you are uncomfortable walking through it."

I remember speaking to Deb about these issues, about the role of spirituality in medicine, and she was literally glowing with excitement. She was a professor of religion, after all. This was her bailiwick. I told her that every patient was different, if one looked deeply enough, and that I was shaped by each encounter. Every conversation was a chance to grow and to redefine myself, not only as a doctor, but as a human being. To know another person, to *really* know them, you need to see the world through their eyes. If you manage it, the world becomes that much larger, and that much more interesting.

It was during this period, with my marriage behind me and as a result of my friendship with Deb, that I began to focus more seriously on questions of religion, spirit, and faith in the face of cancer. During the fellowship, with so many basics to learn, these issues took a backseat. But I had always been affected by my conversations with my patients, and I knew I wasn't alone. Now, with a little time to reflect on this aspect of the practice, I wanted to know what others knew, wanted to feel what they felt, wanted—above all else—to *learn*.

At one point, I put together a five-page survey and asked my fellow physicians to complete it. I was sure there was a link between a doctor's fear of, and discomfort with, death, and the choices he or she made with and for his or her dying patients. Why, for example, would a doctor keep a patient on chemotherapy long after it had stopped helping? Was it because he didn't want to talk about the inevitable? Didn't want to admit, to himself or to his patient, that there was really nothing more he could do?

This made no sense. In the face of cancer, mortality is the everyday question.

As Deb noted, "Cancer brings the threat of chaos into the patient's world, raises the specter of undeserved and incomprehensible human suffering, and introduces death and the demonic." If a patient could not talk openly about these things with her doctor, to whom could she turn? I felt that these conversations needed to be central to our relationships with our patients, because, in the end, that human connection was all that remained.

One afternoon at the county hospital, I found myself in a crowded ward, talking to one of my dying patients about her rapidly diminishing options. In the middle of our conversation, the woman in the neighboring bed suddenly burst into tears. I excused myself for a moment and went to see if there was anything I could do to comfort her. "I'm sorry," she said, trying to get her crying under control. "I couldn't help but overhear, and I know I'm going to die, too, but I'm just not ready to face it."

I had another patient, an elderly woman with late-stage ovarian cancer who was beyond help. "Your cancer is very advanced," I told her. "I don't think additional treatment is going to give you the life you are looking for."

"I imagined as much," she said, then turned to look at her husband, to whom she'd been married for forty years. "But I wanted to make sure that I tried everything possible."

She was doing it for *him*. It was as clear as day. She wanted him to know that she had done everything she could to stay alive, and that there was nothing left to do—that it was time to let go.

Another patient, a black woman, always smiling, good-natured, full of energy. She had recurrent cervical cancer, but she was hanging on. "Where is my little white girl?" she'd holler when she saw me coming, laughing. I sat with her and listened to her talk about her children, her friends, the good people at her church.

"Your whole life seems to be about other people," I said.

"It is," she said, beaming. "I like doing things for others. Makes me feel good about myself."

She asked me about my life, too. When I told her I was divorced, with a young daughter, she asked me to show her a picture of my daughter, and I brought one the following day.

"That's a beautiful girl," she said. "Mind if I hold on to this picture?"

"Not at all," I said.

"When you get home, you make sure you tell little Jessica that her black grandmother is thinking of her, and that she says hello!"

"I definitely will," I told her.

Her energy kept her alive long after her body was ready to quit. Then one day a close friend of hers was killed in a car accident, and she went into a tailspin.

"I'm tired," she said. "I don't think I can hang on anymore. Maybe it's best if I join my friend. We'll get to know heaven together."

I still think about her from time to time. Helping others had given her life meaning, and it had given her the will to go on. Then a close friend died in a car accident and she decided that she'd had enough. Why? What had tipped the scales? This was a deeply spiritual woman, and God definitely played a part in her life, but now it was time to go. Did she feel she could no longer do anything for anyone? Had her life on earth lost its meaning? Spirituality could be about religion, certainly, but at the end of the day maybe it was ultimately about *meaning*.

I had another patient whose cancer was complicated by the crippling effects of rheumatoid arthritis. "I can't help but wonder what I did to deserve this," she told me.

There was nothing I could say to calm her down, and she died angry. I viewed her death as a failed end-of-life experience.

I treated a woman in her forties in the late stages of recurrent cervical cancer. She had a thirteen-year-old son, and she was destroyed by the knowledge that she wasn't going to be around to watch him grow up. There wasn't much hope, and I didn't want her to suffer needlessly. "I think you might be more comfortable in hospice," I suggested.

When her sister found out about that conversation, she was livid. "You're giving up on her!" she told me. "By suggesting hospice, you're telling her there's nothing more you can do!"

It was true that I could do nothing further to treat her cancer, but I wasn't giving up on her—I was simply helping her manage her situation in the best way I knew how. The sister didn't see it that way, and she went to patient advocacy and complained about me: "Dr. Ramondetta is giving up!"

That was hurtful to me. I thought I had done everything I could for my patient, but her family simply wasn't prepared to face the truth.

The next day, my patient decided she wanted to continue treatment.

Treatment made no sense. It might extend her life by a few weeks, but every day would be worse than the preceding one. I went to see her every day, and I would sit by her bed and listen. She talked mostly about her son, and about all the big plans she had had—about the "lifetime of memories" she had hoped to create for him to take into adulthood. "I miss him already," she said.

"I know," I said. And I did. I had a daughter. I could only imagine what it would be like to be told that I wouldn't be around to see her grow up.

"I don't know what to do," she said.

"You know," I said. "I have this vision of you floating in the center of this room, and there are people around you—your son, your sister, other relatives—that are making your decisions for you, or simply coloring the decisions you need to make. But I want you to think about the *quality* of the time you have left. I want you to think hard about how you want to live the life that's left to you."

A few days later, when I came in the room, she reached for my hand before I'd even reached the side of her bed. "Dr. R, I want to thank you for coming and talking to me so often. I know you have many other patients, and it means a lot to me. I think you're right. I don't want to end up on life support, like that poor woman Terry Schiavo, with my family trying to decide whether to keep me alive or not. I need to make this decision for myself, and I've made it. I'm ready to go home. I want to spend the time I have left with my son."

Dying isn't really about "giving up." As death gets closer,

you have to shift your goals. If you only have a little time left, and you spend it struggling to live, that's not going to make for much of a final chapter. You should be focusing on life. On the survivors. On the people you are leaving behind. On your children and grandchildren.

Rafael Campo, a doctor and poet, often talks about death. In one poem, he writes, ". . . more dying waits/ . . . for me . . . / Same hunger . . . Same face . . . / As I examine them, I find the tomb/ Toward which they lead. I know it is my own."

No matter what you believe, we all end up in the same place. Death is the Great Equalizer. That is one of life's great ironies. I see patients of great intrinsic faith and think, "I want what they have." But these patients often have little else. They are often women who are defined as "underserved" or "indigent." They might be black, Hispanic, Baptist, Catholic, but, if they believe, they generally go with peace of mind. They seem to feel that this—the illness—is part of God's plan, and that there must be a reason for it, so they don't struggle as much. Let Go and Let God . . . isn't that what some say?

Others convert at the last minute, fear turning them into believers. And still others don't know what to believe, and often ask me what *I* believe. "I believe there's something bigger than us, but I don't know what it is," I tell them. "But I also believe that nobody is micromanaging our lives, and that sometimes things happen for which there is no discernible reason."

These conversations led, inevitably, to questions about choices. Sometimes my patients leave the decisions up to me, and I wonder if that's what they really want—and even if it's wise. I don't want them to think that I have the power to alter their fate, but I do want them to know that I care, and that it is an honor to be part of their cancer journey.

When my time comes, I will choose a physician who genuinely cares. I'm not sure I'll have peace of mind, or that I'll be able to give up my need for control, which can be formidable, but I want to be in the presence of a doctor who knows me as more than a patient—who has taken the time to connect with the real me. I'm sure I'll have plenty of questions of my own, and some of them will be the same questions I've been asking myself for as long as I can remember: Is there anything out there? What does a human life amount to? What has *my* life meant?

I may not have the answers to these questions, but I'm not going to wait till the end to ask them—I'm going to be asking my whole life. I don't think there's anything more profound than mortality, my own and that of my patients. Thinking about death, and helping people and families face death, is a big part of who I am and what I do.

Learning about dying was teaching me a little something about living.

5

THE ART OF DYING

Several weeks after the BMT, when Deb was feeling better, we went to a local production of *Carmen,* my very first opera. We were very elegantly dressed, and I was wearing high heels, but not Deb—she didn't believe in high heels. After the opera, we walked to a Cuban restaurant and sat in the patio, on very cushy seats, surrounded by reddish curtains that billowed in the breeze.

I tried to be attentive—Was Deb tired? Did she feel well enough to eat? Did she want to cut the evening short?—but Deb waved off my concerns. "Enough about me," she said, laughing. "Let's talk about you."

As I said, Deb wasn't interested in everyone, but when she was interested it was immediately apparent.

. . .

I remain curious about Lois's take on the world. I am invariably surprised by what she has to say, and I find her professional life extraordinary in its engagement with the human drama—and in the degree of responsibility she is willing to shoulder to do her work well. And she does her work marvelously well. Respected by all, feared by some, and greatly beloved by her patients, she carries the lives of these women with an intensity that tires me even as I write about it.

I've mentioned this before, but professionally I have winged it and sometimes misquoted sources in lecture. And no one died. I had the margin to go into class the following week and set it straight. In my academic work on an obscure first-century Alexandrian Jew named Philo, I have made obscure arguments that may have a minimal impact on the ways in which current scholarship assesses the work of this contemporary of Jesus. I have had students say that I have helped them understand the religious texts of traditions not their own and others who have said that I have helped them learn to write. Both accomplishments are good. But no one has thanked me for saving her life or expressed her gratitude to me for seeing her through illness and staying with her until the bitter end. I have cancer, but I could not do cancer work. The weight of the responsibilities involved in doing oncology far exceeds my strengths, and my weaknesses are too numerous to name.

Lois takes it all on and holds herself to a standard of excellence that most physicians cannot imagine. I know that she wakes in the middle of the night, worried about particularly precarious patients.

Lois is almost thirteen years younger than me, and I have the Ph.D., but she is the real doctor in the house. Women often think of friendship as a confessional, the site where all secrets are told and all hair comes down. This is not initially what brought us together or what constitutes the stuff of our relationship. My old friend Neysa Turner, now more than eighty and living outside of Victoria, British Columbia, said of Giles, immediately before I married him, that I "would never be bored." Friendships like marriages are really all about the conversation. Will you find what he or she has to say interesting in a year or in twenty?

From time to time, during her frequent visits to Houston, Deb would come to my house for dinner.

I remember one night in particular, because Elsa was out and Jessica refused to go to bed unless I went with her. She was sitting at the top of the stairs, crying fake tears, until finally Deb couldn't take it anymore. "Don't be ridiculous, Jessie," she said. "Your mother and I are talking. It's time to go to bed. Give her a break."

It was harsh, but it worked, and I know Deb was only looking out for me. Still, I wasn't long past the divorce, and I was dealing with my maternal guilt by letting Jessie sleep in bed with me. It was really my own fault, I guess. I had created a habit that Jessica found hard to break, a habit designed, in part, to help me deal with my own issues. I was without a husband, after all, and I felt very much alone. In fact, after eleven years of postgraduate training, I was completely on my own for the first time, and this even extended to my professional life: I was no longer a fellow-in-training but the person responsible for my patients' medical care.

So, yes—it was a little overwhelming.

At the end of the day, I had my baby to come home to, and when I was with her I felt less alone. But even that was the case only half the time. Ross and I had agreed to share custody, and we honored the agreement. I missed her terribly when she was not with me. At night, I fell asleep in front of the TV, watching movies and trying not to ache for her, and early the next morning I'd be jogging through the neighboring streets, sweating out my frustrations. I remember thinking, *I expected my life to turn out like a fairy tale, and it didn't.*

It was around then that I decided to try to prepare Jessica for the Real World. I thought a good first step would be to avoid any stories with happy endings. Snow White certainly fit the bill. *Letting a stranger into your house!* How dumb is that? As for Cinderella, she had no problem getting on her hands and knees to scrub floors, while her sisters were out partying—where was her self-respect? I found that I preferred books like *The Paper Bag Princess*, by Robert Munsch and Michael Martchenko, which didn't have a traditional happy ending: The Princess has plenty of good reasons to dump the guy, and she does. And she isn't even *thinking* of taking him back. Now that's an ending.

Throughout that first postdivorce year, I also began to notice that certain items in the house evoked negative feelings. Photographs. Mementos. Trinkets we'd collected in the course of the marriage. I didn't want to be defined by any of those objects, so one by one I began getting rid of them.

I was still going to my once-a-week salsa class and enjoying the company of the pleasant, nonthreatening men I met on the dance floor—and left on the dance floor. Dancing made me feel sexy and confident, and I was so focused on the moves that I had little time to dwell on Jessica or on work. It felt *good* to be there. I started feeling more like a woman, and less like the loser character in a bad fairy tale.

On the drive home from salsa class, however, I became Lois again—a single mother with the usual single-mother worries: Will my child be okay? Will I ever fall in love again? And if I do, how will I know he's The One? By the time I crawled into bed, the small thoughts gave way to the big, existential questions—*Who am I? Where am I going? What does it all mean?*—questions that, in my case, predated puberty.

My religious upbringing, though essentially Jewish, was significantly influenced by my father's Catholic upbringing. In other words, I was confused. But I finally decided it was time to become unconfused, and I made Jessica part of the adventure. We went to a Catholic mass, to a local temple, and, finally, to a Unitarian church. I found this last place the most welcoming, and I found the congregation gentle and all-inclusive. I've never understood why so many religions define themselves by excluding people, and this place made me feel accepted from the moment I'd walked through its doors.

I remember telling Deb, "It's funny. My Jewish friends

often call me a MOT [Member of the Tribe], despite my Italian name. But I don't really *feel* like a MOT."

Deb told me that Giles had converted to Judaism after they were married, the culmination of a spiritual journey begun long before they met, and one which was reflected in some of his writing. Deb believed that his conversion also reflected his desire at a certain moment in her illness to do something symbolic for their family. She said that he had said, "I may not be a good Jew, but I'm a happy Jew."

This made me think about happiness in general, and how it differed from person to person, and that, in turn, got me talking to Deb about a new, troubling patient—a young woman with cervical cancer. She had developed a fistula, creating an unnatural connection between two parts of her body. We were able to get the cancer, but in the course of the treatment her bowel had become connected to her vagina, and fluids and other substances that nature intended to stay in the bowel area were seeping instead into her vagina. Honestly—it is hard to imagine anything worse. Finally, I fixed the problem by taking her into surgery and rerouting the misguided bowel loop. She was so grateful that she wept. "Thank you," she said. "Thank you, thank you, thank you! You have made me very happy." That's all it took. That, and the knowledge that she still had many Sundays ahead of her, so she could go to church to sing and pray and socialize. For her, this was happiness.

"It makes me wonder, 'What the hell am I complaining about?'" I told Deb.

"I know what you mean," she said. "It's all about perspective, and none of us is very good at it."

In March, Deb was well enough to go home. She asked me to come visit her in California. One of the other doctors found this amusing. "Lois isn't laid back enough for California," he said, tickled pink at his own observation. He was right. I definitely have control issues, and I will be the first to admit that I'm nowhere near as easygoing as I'd like to be. My mother once gave me a copy of *Who Moved My Cheese?*, the book by Spencer Johnson. It is designed for people who don't deal well with change, and that was me all the way—Lois the Inflexible. But I was working on it. And, as with everything else, I was learning.

From the moment Deb left, I missed her horribly. It was a palpable absence. I would call her from the car on my way home, and we'd catch up. She was feeling well, she told me, and was being deluged with cancer questions by friends, friends of friends, and friends of those friends.

As one might imagine, longevity in cancer care has given me a kind of notoriety, and people often call me for advice and medical referrals. This is work I am very happy to do, and I divide my narrative advice into three parts. The first concerns the Internet: Stay off of it. On ovarian cancer, all the news is bad. As for protocols and procedures, the ill, or at least the first-time ill, are not in a position to make judgments about the appropriateness of one course of treatment over another.

The second involves the kind of care one should seek. Go to a research hospital, a hospital affiliated with the teaching and training of medical and surgical oncologists. Amazing advances have occurred over the last forty years in cancer care, and they invariably start in these university settings. Other hospitals are doubtless doing their best, but, generally speaking, community oncologists cannot be as aggressive as physicians working in a university setting. This is another way of saying, "Get the best care you can." All physicians want their patients to get well, but some of them are better at medicine than others—and some are better equipped for it.

Finally, try to enjoy the life you have before you. A friend, Fran Lantz, told me after five years in chemotherapy, a colostomy, more surgeries, and worse, "Enjoy your chemotherapy." She had run through all the available chemotherapy options and had even tried some phase I clinical trials. Despite all of this, it was just about over. In Fran's universe, chemotherapy was a good thing, and one should enjoy it accordingly. I am trying.

I have also had the extraordinarily good fortune to have Dr. Margaret Sun as my oncologist in Santa Barbara. To say I love Dr. Sun misses the point. She is inscribed in my heart. Even when I don't see her, I see her in my imagination. She has taken exquisite care of me since I was diagnosed and has worked with the oncologists at M. D. Anderson, to the benefit of both, I imagine. She engages cancer both as a disease and as a molecular puzzle. Blazingly smart, she is a bit younger than I am and has a family that includes a husband and four beautiful children. I am a grateful patient, and I have offered my academic services to her kids. They generally come with lunch, but one memorable afternoon I gave an hour-and-a-half lecture on the origins of the Palestinian-Israeli problem to Dr. Sun's daughter, Jenny, who is a freshman in college. How did she sit through it? I don't know, but I had no choice but to listen to myself speak: I was hooked up and receiving a new drug, avastin, through infusion.

When I realized that cancer care and chemotherapy would be part of my life until I died, I changed my attitude toward it. I now schedule my time with Dr. Sun in the early afternoon and arrive with lunch for her, her assistant, and her daughter—if she happens to be working in the office on the day of the appointment. We have a quick meal together—I eat soup—and then Dr. Sun readies me for chemotherapy. It involves accessing the Port-o-Cath in my chest, drawing blood, and waiting while the blood is evaluated. If all the variables are satisfactory, the infusion begins.

If I am very lucky, Jenny will come in and tell me about her life and times. Late in the afternoon, Dr. Sun may sit with me and we can discuss the world, the crisis in American health care, and the issues related to parenting and to being married. She is a woman and now a friend that I would not have met apart from ovarian cancer, and I am better for having her in my life. One Christmas I thanked her for making my cancer journey such a pleasure. And she knew what I meant. It has not been a pleasure, but it has been easier for me because she has cared for me and brought me into the orbit of her world.

Much later, I learned that Dr. Sun had a very small practice, and that this was by design. Apparently, shortly after one of her patients died, she read the woman's obituary in the local newspaper, and she was astonished by all the things she didn't know about her. This saddened her, and she vowed never to be in that position again. From that day forth, she cared for only as many patients as she could handle—as many patients as she could get to know.

"She's an oncologist who makes house calls," Deb told me. "You'll meet her. You'll like her. She is interesting and interested."

Deb always ended our conversations by saying, "We have a room for you and Jessie in our house. Come visit!"

Sundays I would always try to do something special with Jessie. The zoo, the local parks, a children's museum, a train ride, finger painting. Whenever we were in the car, driving to our next adventure, we would invariably listen to a local DJ known to his fans as the Big Boss Man of the Blues. Traditionally, blues music is thought to be sad and plaintive, but this DJ—Nuri Nuri—somehow managed to put a positive spin on it.

That year, 2001, my first year as a single mom, Elsa took Jessica and me out for dinner on my birthday. She had become a real friend by this time. Her brother joined us, and the four of us had a great time. We went to a Mexican restaurant and the mariachis came to the table and sang happy birthday. It was all wonderfully silly, and I managed not to cry.

Elsa was a real rock in our lives. One of her favorite books was *The Celestine Prophecy,* which she read in Spanish. I picked up an English version once—it's about spirituality,

and the many "insights" that lead people to a higher plane—
but it was a little too New Age for me, and I never finished
it. Elsa also loved Spanish soap operas. Sometimes I'd come
home and find her and Jessie glued to the television set, both
of them entranced. I'm not sure Jessie understood what she
was seeing, but she certainly seemed to find it interesting.

In June, at the end of my first year as an attending physician, I decided to take Deb up on her invitation, and I flew out
to California with Jessica.

She and Giles were living in Santa Barbara at the time, in
a spacious older house with a big backyard and a swimming
pool. The house itself was full of eclectic art: African masks
and knitted tribal costumes, American folk art and abstracts
that Deb had painted. And there were books, of course, books
everywhere, *mountains* of books.

From the moment we arrived, Jessica and I felt completely
at home. It was like going on vacation with a tiny girlfriend.

I must say, we were crazy about California. I may not be
the most laid back person on the planet, but I loved riding
around in Deb's "BMW/BMT Freedom Car," and I especially
loved the sun and the salty air, whether at the beach or just
lounging around the pool at their house.

Jessica couldn't get enough of Sheba, the family mastiff.
Sheba was three times my daughter's size, but she still let Jessica think she was in charge. She also liked the family cat,
Maxx, which had wildly deformed front legs but lived his life
completely unaware of any "disability."

One day, on her way to yoga, Deb dropped me at the office

of a local man who practiced alternative medicine. "He has helped me through some of the more painful parts of my cancer journey," she said.

The man was very soft-spoken, and his clinic was very peaceful—all done up in wood and bamboo. He made me soak in a very hot hot-tub just before my massage.

I got back to the house, wonderfully sore in every muscle, to find Jessica and Deb in the living room, dancing to Shakira. The two of them had grown very close on that short trip. After dancing, they picked oranges in the yard and made fresh orange juice for all of us.

After we put Jessie to bed, Deb made hot tea and we sat outside, near the pool.

"A cup of tea is a joy forever," she said.

"You look good," I said.

"I'm trying to align myself with the living," she replied. "I don't want to think about death. I'm in remission. I'm happy to be alive. I have my children back and I'm home with my darling husband. What more can a girl ask?"

The next night, we went salsa dancing with Deb's friend Genevieve. Giles stayed home with Jessica and proved to be an excellent sitter.

We also did plenty of shopping in Santa Barbara, which was very dangerous for me. Deb could do serious damage to the family pocketbook in a very short amount of time, whether she was at Neiman Marcus or at one of the many quaint stores in downtown Santa Barbara. In the space of a few hours, as we made our way from store to store, she bought a Hindu statue, an Indian carving, and a pair of big African gold hoop earrings.

We shopped when she was in Houston, too. I introduced her to a store called the Blue Hand, which had a wonderfully eclectic collection: Mexican Day of the Dead stuff, African masks, Buddhas in every imaginable shape and size, and, of course, plenty of hands. One of the hands, made of papier-mâché, was supposed to be the hand of Jesus, and it had figures of various saints and apostles sitting lengthwise atop the fingers. Deb took my hand. "Lois," she commanded, "you have to buy that."

Deb knew that I was interested in hands. We had often talked about the healing power of touch at bedside, and about the way people connect and comfort each other by reaching out with their hands. I bought the Jesus hand, and it was the first hand in what was to become, over the years, a fairly extensive collection. I am now the proud owner of hands from all over the world. It seems that most faiths ascribe great power to hands and to human touch—Jews, Catholics, Muslims, Hindus, Buddhists, etc.—and I'm always looking out for new and unusual examples. My very favorite, though, was a gift from Deb: It is a ceramic surgical glove, which she painted herself, that represents the hand of a surgeon, *my* hand. And the truth is, my hands play an unusually important role in my surgery. Many surgeons rely primarily on surgical instruments, slowly dissecting and probing, but I often use my fingers—what others call my "Ramondettas"—to make my way around. It makes me feel closer to my patients, more connected, better informed.

When Deb and I returned from our little shopping expedition, loaded with things, Giles's eyes went wide. "So I spent a little money!" Deb said. "What's the big deal? It's not like I'm planning for retirement."

Giles just shook his head, smiling.

A few days later, Jessica and I left Santa Barbara and went to visit friends in Los Angeles. What I remember most about that leg of the trip was going to the beach in Venice and digging for sand crabs. Jessica was ecstatic. The tiny crabs would scurry up and down her arms, trying to escape, and she was laughing so hard she had trouble catching her breath.

We ended our trip with a visit to Disneyland, a happy place where every princess was lucky enough to find her prince. I was still in my anti-fairy-tale phase, but I kept my thoughts to myself and let Jessica enjoy herself with Cinderella, Sleeping Beauty, and—her very favorite—Ariel.

Shortly after we got back to Houston, and to life at M. D. Anderson, my parents came to visit again. I took them to a German beer garden that weekend, to a party that was being sponsored by a local radio station, and by one of its weekend DJs—Nuri Nuri, the Big Boss Man of the Blues. I had been listening to him ever since I'd moved to Houston, and I went over and introduced myself.

"I know you," I said. "I'm a regular listener!"

"Oh, thank you, and thanks for listening," he said.

We talked for a minute and then he had to get back to

work, so Jessica and I went off to dance a little, but when he took a break he came by our table and bought me a beer and we chatted briefly. It turned out that Nuri was a systems analyst who had worked at M. D. Anderson for ten years, coordinating the computer training department and launching an online training program for the Cancer Center. He was also an accomplished bass player, however, and had been a volunteer radio DJ at Pacifica Public Radio for fifteen years, and music was his passion. When he found out I was divorced, we kept in touch by e-mail, and a few weeks later he asked me out. I wondered if some of that Disney magic had rubbed off on me, and whether I'd been wrong to banish fairy tales from our home.

We met one cold Sunday at a coffee shop near his radio station, right after his show, and we talked all afternoon and into the evening while sitting outside, our leather jackets zipped tight. I learned that Nuri was Palestinian. He was born in Jerusalem, but had come to the United States in his late teens to complete his college education, and had liked it so much that he had stayed and become a U.S. citizen. In Houston, where he'd settled, he was quite the local celebrity. Every so often, someone would interrupt our conversation by calling out to him: "Nuri Nuri! The Big Boss Man of the Blues! I'm a big fan."

He took time to thank everyone, and he had a wonderful, gentle smile. I was already taken with him.

When I got home, I e-mailed Deb to tell her about this unusual, exotic man. She wrote back, clearly happy for me, but also a tad cautious: "Lois dear, crosscultural romance is a very difficult business." Maybe she was right—I was a Jew, albeit a confused Jew, and he was a Palestinian—but I was intrigued and didn't want to be talked out of it. So I dealt with it by changing the subject: "Deb, I have been thinking about doing a paper about the 'art of dying' for one of the medical journals. With your background in religion, I think you would be the perfect co-author. What do you think?"

"I think you are brilliant!" she replied. "Absolutely!"

I had been thinking about the topic for a very long time. A few days later, eager to get going, I slipped into Academic Mode and sent Deb a few paragraphs.

Shortly after, not having heard back from Deb, I became my impatient self again and wrote:

> Just wondering—have you gotten a chance to look at what I sent you?
>
> Do you know of any books that look at the way people of different religions approach "cancer"? Do you think we could talk more? I am really interested also in getting more education on the subject of ethics and oncology (certainly I have more time than I know what to do with—kidding!). However, I would like to talk with you a little on where you think this interest could be directed.

I also had time to write about my blossoming romance with Nuri, which had already resulted in two more dates:

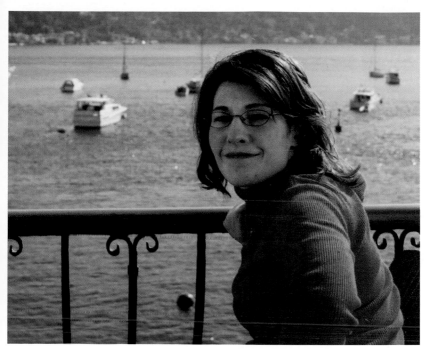

Lois Ramondetta, 2004.

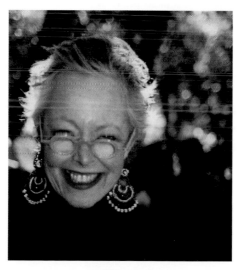

Deborah Rose Sills, 2005.

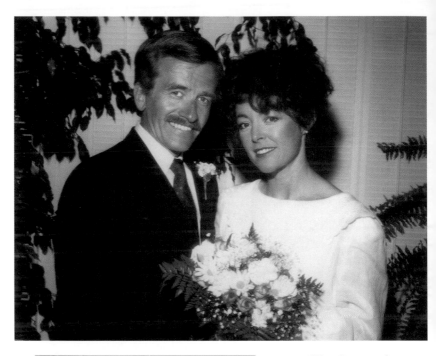

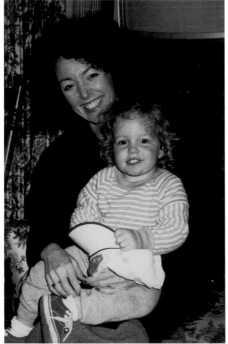

above: *Giles Gunn and Deborah on their wedding day, July 9, 1983.*

left: *Deborah and Abigail Rose Gunn in Gainesville, Florida, 1985.* (Giles Gunn)

facing page, top: *Deborah on the banks of the James River in Williamsburg, Virginia, 1984.* (Giles Gunn)

facing page, bottom: *Deborah and Abby in Paris on Abby's ninth birthday, June 9, 1993.* (Giles Gunn)

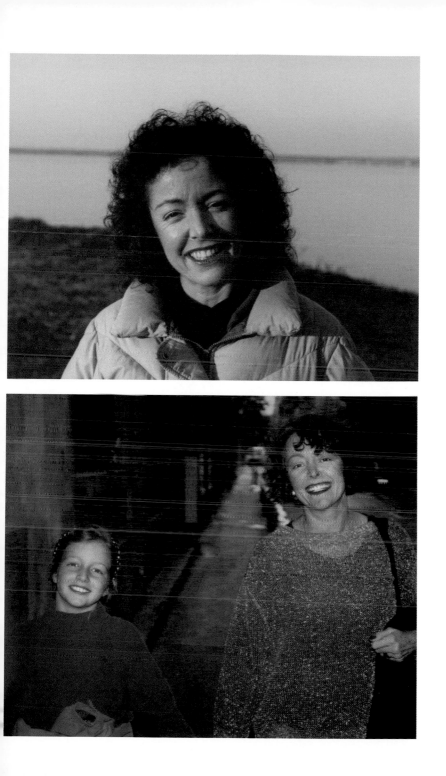

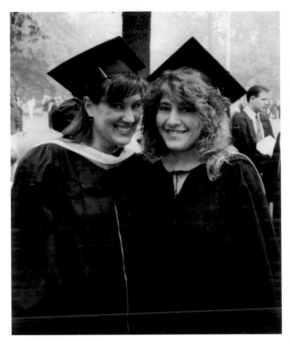

Ellen (Bonner) Oliver and Lois on their graduation day from Emory University, 1989.

Lois with her parents, June and Paul Ramondetta, on her graduation from the University of Medicine and Dentistry of New Jersey (Rutgers), 1993.

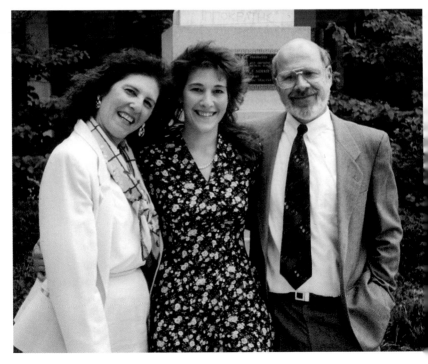

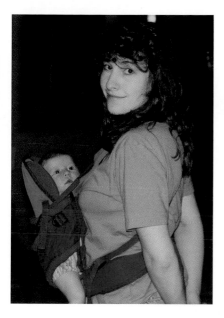

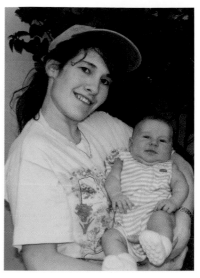

Lois and baby Jessica, 1997.

above: *Lois and baby Jessica Bea during Lois's last year of residency in obstetrics/gynecology at Thomas Jefferson University in Philadelphia, 1997.*

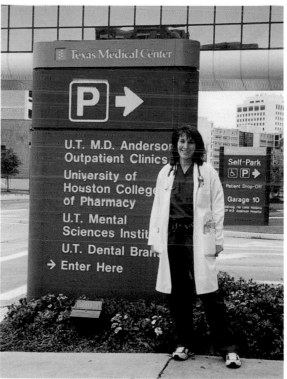

Lois during the last year of her fellowship at M. D. Anderson Cancer Center, 2000.

(Paul and June Ramondetta)

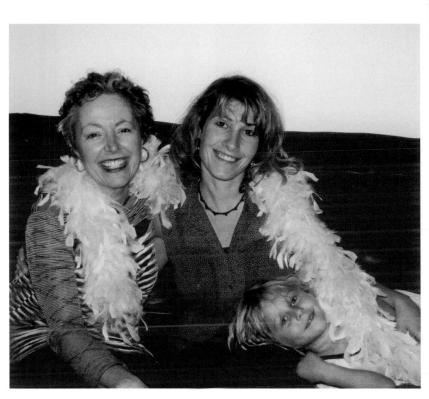

Deborah, Jessica, and Lois at Lois's house in Texas, 2000.

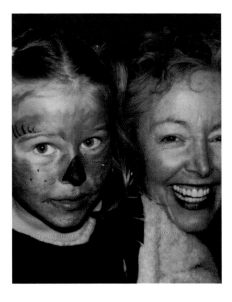

Deborah with Jessica, after watching Jessica perform in The Lion King, *2000.*

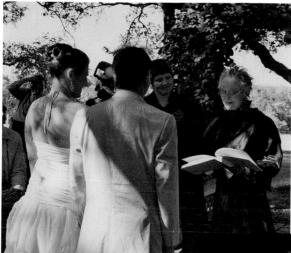

Deborah giving the sermon at Lois and Nuri A. Nuri's wedding, April 30, 2005.

Deborah and Lois, laughing on Lois's wedding day.

Nuri and Lois on their wedding day.

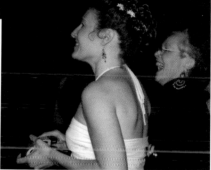

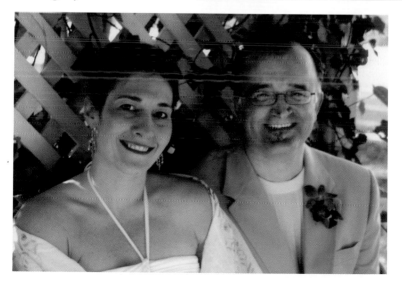

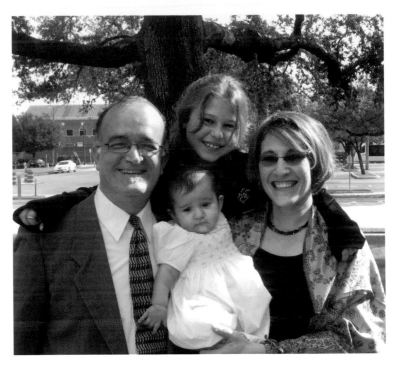

Nuri, Jessica, Leila, and Lois, December 2006.

Lois and Nuri, June 2007.

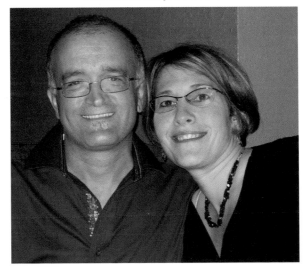

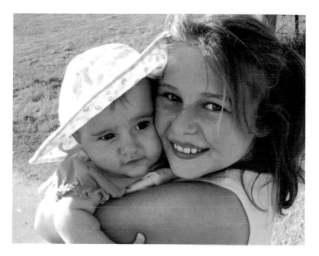

Leila Rose and Jessica Bea, November 2006.

*Lois and Leila, upon a surprise visit from Nuri at
M. D. Anderson, August 2007.*

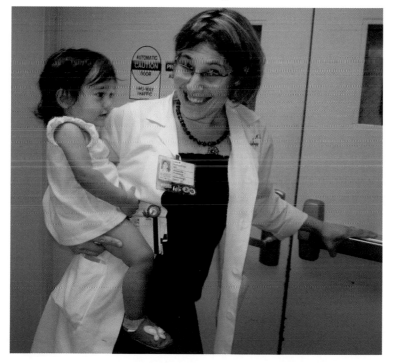

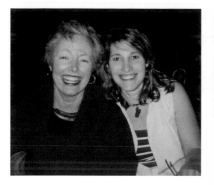

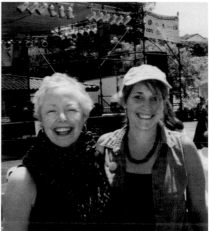

above: *Deborah and Lois, Houston 2001.*

above right: *Deborah and Lois at a Santa Barbara fair, 2001.*

right: *Deborah and Lois on their way to salsa in Santa Barbara, 2001.*

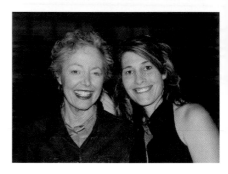

below: *Deborah and Lois at the Turkish bath in Paris, 2004.*

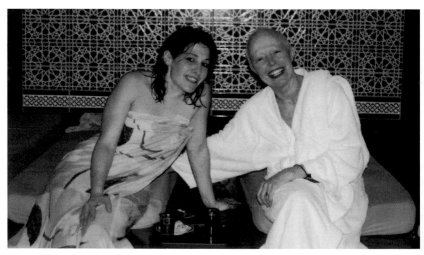

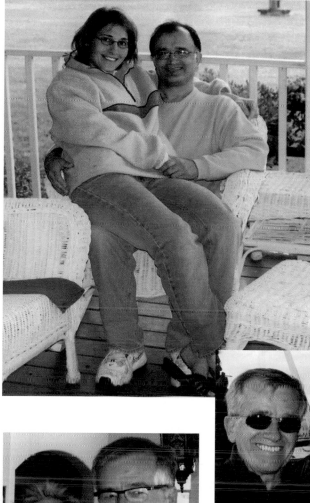

Lois and Nuri on the porch of Mariposa Ranch in Brenham, Texas, during their wedding weekend, 2005.

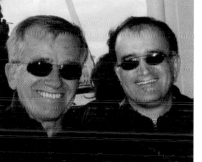

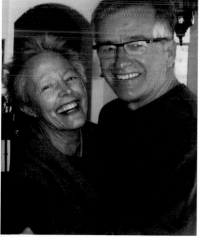

above: *Giles and Nuri on a ferry in Istanbul, Turkey, 2004.*

left: *Deborah and Giles dancing in Lois and Nuri's home, January 2006.*

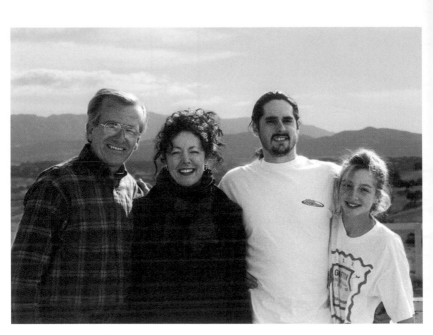

*Giles, Deborah, Adam, and Abby on the ranch
in Los Olivos, California, 1995.*

*Giles, Adam, Abby, and Deborah taking some time in the sun,
Ventura, California, spring 2006.*

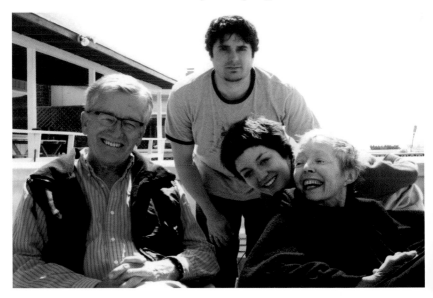

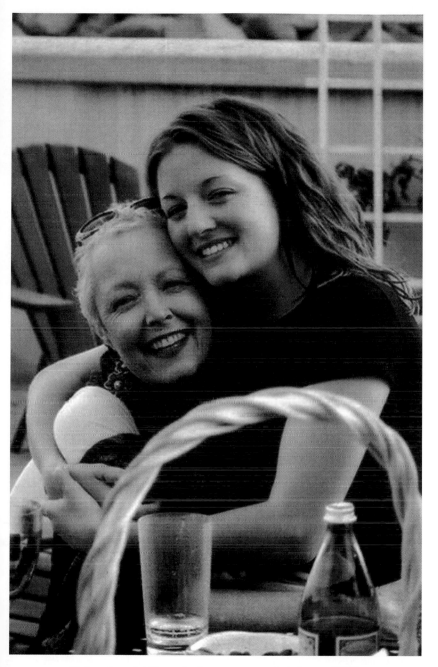

Deborah and Abby enjoying a party at their home, 2003.
(Giles Gunn)

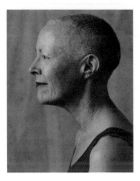

above: *Deborah after finishing the first round of chemotherapy treatments, Santa Barbara, California, 1998.*

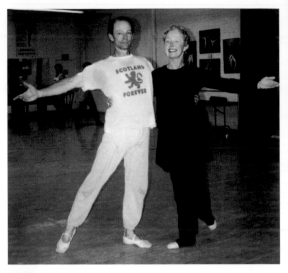

above: *Deborah with Gary McKenzie, a cofounder and principal dancer at State Street Ballet, Santa Barbara, California, 2001.*

left: *Deborah playing violin.*

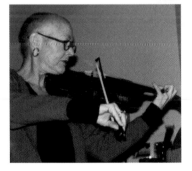

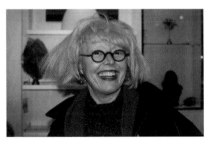

above: *Deborah trying on wigs at Le Bon Marche on Lois and Deborah's first night together in Paris, 2004.* (Lois Ramondetta)

left: *Giles and Deb dancing in Lois and Nuri's home to a dedication Nuri made to them via the radio on his* Sunday Blues Brunch *show (KPFT 90.1) the same morning that Deborah received the news that she now also had a rare form of leukemia, Houston, Texas, 2006.* (Lois Ramondetta)

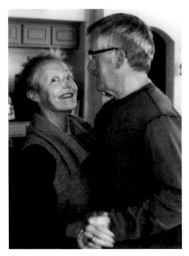

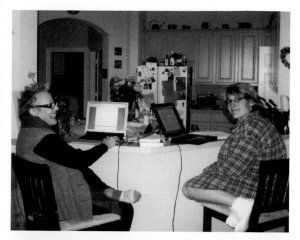

left: *Lois and Deborah working hard on the book while listening to Odetta, as Nuri took photos over Lois's protests, insisting that these were moments they "didn't want to forget."* (Nuri Akram Nuri)

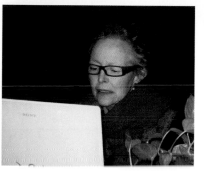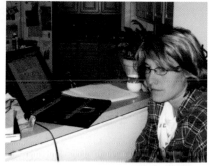

above, left and right: *Deborah and Lois at work writing* The Light Within, *as they listen to Odetta singing "This Little Light of Mine," January 2006.*

right: *Deborah and Lois writing the book together over breakfast in Istanbul, Turkey, 2004.*

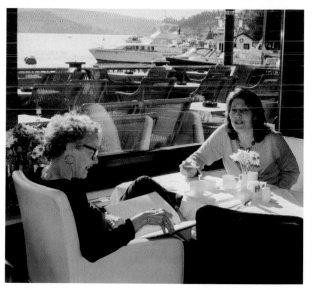

Deborah a year before her diagnosis, the Dingle Peninsula, Republic of Ireland, summer 1996. (Giles Gunn)

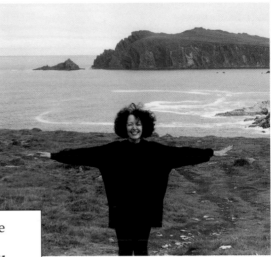

Memorial Service
for
Deborah Rose Sills

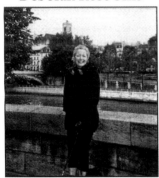

May 6, 2006
Unitarian Society
Santa Barbara, California

The front cover of the program for the memorial service for Deborah Rose Sills, May 2006.

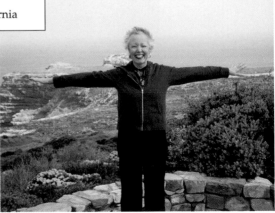

Deborah standing on the Cape of Good Hope, South Africa, summer 2002.
(Giles Gunn)

I went out with Nuri last night, and—Palestinian or not—it seems his background is very similar to mine. Certainly he is a talker and I get the sense the two groups (Israelis and Palestinians) have a lot more in common than the rest of the world thinks. He actually went to high school in an American-Quaker school in Palestine and then came here for college. He is 43 so I think he has been here for 20+ years. Still very connected to his culture . . . many Arabic friends. Anyway—I do enjoy him—very interesting man.

We went for sushi and a great coffee bar with cool jazz music last night and had a great time. I would like you to meet him. Love ya—Lois

Deb wrote back to tell me that she was excited about meeting him, too. She also filled me in on other details of her life, all of them non-medical. The big news was that she and Giles were thinking of buying a house on the beach, which she said was beyond their means, but which they had both fallen in love with. She also reported, with justifiable pride, that Giles would be going to the University of Alabama at Tuscaloosa shortly to deliver the annual Martin Luther King, Jr., Memorial Lecture. "He's the first white guy to do it," she noted.

In the weeks ahead, we worked on the paper, sending it back and forth, listening to each other's suggestions, making changes. She also wrote about her ongoing treatment up in Santa Barbara, and about her efforts to live as normal a life as possible:

I have been busy with chemotherapy every week, teaching twice a week, and then the details of daily living. I'm finished teaching on the 16th of May and plan simply to enjoy yoga and dancing for a bit. . . . I've got to take Abby to school now. She debuts as the Queen of England tonight in *A Tale of Two Cities*.

Over the course of the next few weeks—between her chemotherapy and trips to Abby's school and romantic dinners with Giles (and less romantic discussions about the beach house)—Deb was able to concentrate on our paper. We were both very excited about it, since it dealt with a subject we had been talking about almost from the day we'd met—specifically, the relationship between the physician and the patient in the face of terminal illness. As part of our research, we looked at much of the work that had been published on issues related to definitions of spirituality, and at the many ways in which religious or spiritual concerns informed and sometimes even molded the relationships between the patients and their physicians. We also looked at whether there was something specific in, or unique to, the experience of women patients with reproductive cancers, and at the way treating such patients affected physicians and other medical personnel.

The paper was subsequently published in the *Journal of Clinical Oncology*, and it appeared under both our names. It was called "Spirituality and Religion in the 'Art of Dying,'" and it opened as follows: "Oncologists, because of the character of the diseases they treat, find themselves addressing end-of-life concerns with their patients more often than they might prefer."

The paper discussed how a doctor's attitude toward death influenced the way in which end-of-life discussions were managed, and whether his or her discomfort with death influenced decisions regarding treatment—especially when it was clear that continued treatment wasn't going to change the outcome. "Like their patients, physicians must come to terms with the finite character of all human experience," we wrote. "In most cases, it involves at the very least an intimate conversation between patient and physician that can afford both a greater appreciation of the gifts of being alive and a renewable sense of hopefulness about human resiliency. . . . What makes the experience real for the patient is good communication with his or her physician."

In July of 2002, just as Nuri and I were celebrating six months together, he went to Jordan to visit his parents, who had relocated there temporarily. His father was suffering from advanced Alzheimer's, and his mother was caring for him on her own.

Before Nuri left, he asked me to watch his house for him while he was gone. We communicated almost daily via e-mail, but by the third week he had grown a little distant. "Love and kisses to Jessica," he would write.

That's all very well and good, I would think, but what about *me*?

Then I got a terrible e-mail—a *Dear Lois* e-mail. He was

breaking up with me. I was devastated. It seemed his mother didn't approve of me because I was of a different religion. She hadn't told him what to do, but she had raised serious doubts in his mind about our future.

"I love you very much," he wrote, "but my trip back home has made me realize that my life here, despite its freedom, is still heavily tied to traditions and beliefs and as much as I might want to break away from some of these traditions I cannot, not yet. I want to continue to spend time with you although I know you may not be ready to do this if I cannot promise any more than friendship."

He got that part, at least, right. I was incredibly upset. I wrote to tell him that he should look for someone else to take care of his house, and I wrote Deb to tell her what had happened, going so far as to share his e-mail with her.

So much for fairy tales!

She wrote back on July 29, 2002:

Dearest Lois, [. . .]

This hurts and I can imagine why it is you are in some difficulty—however, take a deep breath and begin to think of his note as one twelfth of himself, the part that spends one month a year in the Middle East. Reading it from "the outside," it represents an internal conversation with himself about growing up and the difficulty he has in being honest with his parents about the kind of life he leads in the United States. This may not help you immediately, but it is important for you to see this for what it is—and it is a letter full of confusion, love for you, and fear about the demands for loyalty that his parents [and] his culture are making on him. We all have these factors working on us, and one of the things we need to do is to come to terms with these conflicts—to do what Socrates charged us with doing many moons ago—Know Thyself. This is the stuff of Nuri's dilemma. And interestingly enough this is not really your problem. You are yourself and your friends and colleagues love you for it and respect you for it. It is the stuff that enables you to chew on Jessie's legs with abandon because you know and now she knows that your whole self, without qualification, loves her. There is more to say here and some of it might be best said on the phone. I'll try you later. Be well and get some exercise. Boy, am I crazy about you. Much love, Deb

There were other e-mails about other topics, also related to heartbreak, if a different kind:

Abby is coming home this weekend with a ring in her lip. . . . I guess it is good it is not a nose-ring.

Then my mother was diagnosed with a small bladder cancer, which was successfully dealt with, and Deb wrote asking for news and expressing sympathy:

Being diagnosed with cancer is akin to being hit by a train. Nothing is ever the same afterwards.

On the heels of this, Nuri returned from Amman, but I didn't want to see him. I was deeply hurt and, to be honest, angry. I could understand his obligations to his culture, but here he was, a man in his forties, wanting marriage and kids, but fighting his attraction to me. *Much as I might want to break away from these traditions, I cannot*, he had written. Well, I told myself, fine then; he could figure himself out. I didn't want any part of it.

But it was painful—so painful. We had enjoyed each other so much up until that point. The words "soul mate" had been floated more than once. Even through my anger at him, I was clearheaded enough to admit that the idea that this might not work was deeply painful to both of us, not just to me.

A few weeks later, the musician Keb' Mo' was in town for a concert. We were both big fans, and before everything had fallen apart we'd discussed going together. But with everything that was between us, I assumed our outing was off.

So my breath came out a little unsteady when I opened an e-mail from him saying: "I have 2 tickets to the show tonight and I would love for you to come with me, regardless of what's going on between us."

"I cannot," I wrote back to him. "I want more than anything to go with you—to be with you, but I will not heal with this. Have fun at the concert. I want you to come for me only when you're ready to try (try as long as possible)."

But he was persistent, even while admitting that it was probably a better idea for us not to go together because of our still-tumultuous hopes and feelings. Still, he reasoned, "it might be good for us to be together and start to accept who we are. Please think about it."

Well, anti-fairy-tale or not, my hopes and feelings did eventually play a role. I couldn't help myself; I went to the concert with him. The Keb' Mo' concert was something we both knew we wanted to go to, and we couldn't think of someone we would rather go with. We decided to go, trying to see if we could be "just friends" and not more. It was in a wonderful old theater with red velvet curtains in Conroe, Texas. We sat up close, danced in the aisles, and even got to meet Keb' Mo' backstage. All the while, I secretly hoped Nuri would remember how perfect we were for each other despite our backgrounds.

And that night was the beginning of a new start for us. With time, I think, we realized that we just had so much in common and admired each other so much that we couldn't see our way to ending it because of only the *possibility* of eventual irreconcilable differences.

On October 22, Deb wrote about another topic entirely:

You of course do not know the significance of this day for me, and of course I will tell you. It was five years ago today that I had a hysterectomy (sp?) and learned that

I had ovarian cancer. Looking back, which I am very glad that I can, I wish I had had the original surgery at Anderson—it wouldn't have hurt so much and maybe you guys would have gotten more of it. Nevertheless it has been an extraordinary five years and I count you as one of my real blessings, a surgeon, a wonderful friend, and such an interesting person. My life is so much more full and vibrant with you in it. Hope it goes well today. I'm going to paint a picture, and do some dancing. . . . Lois dear, I'm crazy about you. Much love, Deb

I wrote back:

Well—I am sure this was a big day—so much has changed, I am sure, from what you thought life was all about. This to me is the greatest hoax/misrepresentation given to children. No one ever thinks it is going to be them. You go to school, get a job, get married, have children, get old and die—why is it that people are so unprepared for the inevitable bumps, like cancer and divorce? I guess those that are prepared can be labeled pessimists. On the other hand, I was reading a little about Buddhism and I think (if I understood it) that the thought process about life is more about change and adjusting to changes—being flexible. Lots to talk about here. I also suppose we could just say,"It is all in God's hands," [but] that would be boring: no screaming, yelling, jumping for joy, kicking walls, etc.

I hope you are well! I know you are—I can feel it!

As for Nuri, I am taking it day by day. I truly enjoy the time we spend together but not sure where it is going. He did ask me to meet his best friend in St. Louis, as well as his sister. I am watching myself— sometimes I think it is my duty to enlighten him (or just bounce silly ideas off of him) and vice versa. It is part of the global peace effort!

Days later Deb responded with the following:

Giles sprang a surprise party on me Saturday night, a party celebrating life after five years in the cancer wars. It was wonderful and we all had a great time and I really wish you could have been there. Abby came up from UC Irvine and I was full of feeling and good humor. She seems to be enjoying herself, growing up some and wistful as she recognizes that she has left home in at least the allegorical sense of the term.

Then she wrote again to tell me about having run into an evangelical Christian woman who wanted to know if it was necessary to have a soul to be saved:

The real question is, Saved from what? What she is really interested in is where the dead go after they die and, yes, this is a real question, but who could give us the answer? All most of us get is that there is a long hallway full of light. There must be more going on, don't you think? More later and much love.

Yes, I thought. There must be more going on. Much more. And there was, but not all of it was good.

Long after my second surgery and many chemotherapy varieties, I understood some of the many problems that patients can and often do get into while taking treatment. I was nearly at the end of a series of chemotherapy infusions, Taxol given weekly, in anticipation of returning to M. D. Anderson for a month of radiation therapy. In this instance, I was to have my spleen irradiated because it had become the site where some of the ovarian cancer cells had now lodged. I was to leave for Houston on a Wednesday and was to take my last Taxol treatment on Monday in Dr. Sun's medical office. On the previous Saturday, however, I began to have terrible diarrhea and also started to vomit. I knew what this meant: I needed intravenous liquids so that I would not collapse. This is not a particularly unusual event for cancer patients, but I did feel really badly. Giles drove me to the hospital. I was admitted, given an IV, and so began the hydration. Within a day I was feeling much better. Dr. Sun decided to have the last dose of Taxol delivered to me while I was still in the hospital. This is where the trouble began.

Monday morning the nurses administered the drugs that prepare one for chemotherapy, antinausea, anti-inflammatory drugs, and more saline. Apparently, for safety reasons, the protocol requires that the vein used for chemotherapy must not allow fluid to flow easily into the vein, and must also be a site where the nurse can withdraw blood. The vein that received the prechemotherapy drugs would not oblige the nurses by returning blood. Then the hunt began. Over the course of the next two and a half hours, three different nurses tried to secure a suitable vein on a variety of sites. Sitting in bed, having young women of various types dig around in one's arms with needles, is hard to bear. Sitting still for this required a good deal of discipline. After the last failure, I realized that I was, in a very real sense, free. I was physically unattached to any lines and could walk about without dragging an IV pole with me. And I did just that. I walked out of the hospital. Looking back, I was in a kind of altered state, full of rage and at the same time experiencing a great sense of freedom. I left the hospital, phoned my husband, and headed up to Dr. Margaret Sun's office, a three-block walk from the hospital entrance. Dr. Sun's nurse, Teri, greeted me with a grin and a question: "How did you get out?"

I told her I escaped. Dr. Sun looked at my arms, and because of her great skill and perhaps because I had walked a bit, she inserted a line into my left arm on the first try. She then instructed me to return to the hospital and finish the treatment. Full of self-righteousness, I marched back into the hospital, entered my room on the sixth floor, and informed the nurse that I had solved her Goddamn problem. "Now get the drug and get on with it!" She had her own plans. My departure, or as I understood it, my escape from the hospital, according to protocol, required that I sign a release form, indicating that I had left without the permission of the hospital staff. Before treatment could begin, I was told I must sign a form stipulating that my departure was done without hospital oversight. I refused to sign the release form. I tore it in half and, as I handed it to the nurse, said, "Fuck you."

Another form was printed, and this one was delivered to me by the charge nurse. I repeated the ritual destruction of the form— something out of One Flew Over the Cuckoo's Nest *no doubt*— and said to this lovely woman, "Fuck you, too." I added that I had also solved her Goddamn problem, and that they should get the Goddamn drug and get on with the infusion of the chemotherapy. We were clearly at an impasse.

By this time, Giles was there, observing but deciding not to enter the drama. Not too long after, Dr. Sun arrived. She is an extraordinary woman and an exemplary oncologist. She has been my physician since I started this journey and to simply say that I am grateful for her relentless and lifesaving care, or that I love her, misses the point. All the hospital technicians and nurses know her very well and respect her skill and her thoroughness. The room went quiet when she entered, and just how she repaired the situation, I still don't know. I didn't sign the release. The drug was administered, and I don't remember her saying anything. I did write a note of apology to the nursing staff, and I did leave on Wednesday for M. D. Anderson. It could have been alchemy for all I know, but Dr. Sun managed us all, and we all moved on. Clearly, medicine is not a science. At the difficult times, it is just too human.

6

PAS DE DEUX IN PARIS

Every few months, Deb and Giles came to Houston for follow-ups, always staying at least part of the time with me. My daughter had grown close to Deb, and began to think of her as part of our family.

I also introduced Deb to Nuri, and on our very first night we all went to a local Japanese restaurant together. The conversation was all about the Middle East—very political, even heated at times—but after dinner Deb took me aside and said, "I like this guy."

I liked him, too. We began going on little overnight trips together, and before long—when I was sure things were getting serious—Jessica started coming with us. We would visit rural Texas, saunter through the colorful farmers' markets, ride pontoon boats on Lake Travis, or drive to music concerts.

From time to time, Nuri would take Jessica to the radio station, where he taught her how everything worked, and where she occasionally got to say hello to the fans on the air. She loved that even more than the pontoon boats.

Nuri would also pick her up from camp or school when I was pressed for time, and I'd come home to find them in the house preparing dinner together. Nuri was masterful in front of the stove. He could take a few pieces of chicken, some slices of mango and avocado, and turn them into a truly delicious dinner.

Deb came over one night and was very impressed, with the food and with him. "I like him a lot," she said. "He treats you well."

This was a big issue for her—she felt people didn't treat other people with the kindness and attention they deserved, and she was always pleasantly surprised when they did. "He's a sweetie," she said. "That's what he is. And he's good to you. And he's also broadening your horizons. I mean, look at you— sitting at dinner discussing the Israeli-Palestinian conflict!"

"He is pretty great, isn't he?" I said, unable to keep from smiling.

"He's interesting," she said. "And a good conversationalist. So, yes—I approve."

A few days later, while Deb was still in Houston, I invited her to watch Jessica in a school production of *The Lion King*.

When I found out that Jessie's dad was going to attend with his new fiancée, I was a little nervous, because this would be my very first meeting with her. Deb laughed it off, and suggested that we all get gussied up for the occasion. We did— and we looked really hot—but the fiancée never showed up. I was a little disappointed, to be honest; I had my support team with me, and I was ready to face her. Still, the play more than made up for it.

Deb was effusive in her praise of Jessica's performance, and Jessica couldn't get enough of it.

"You *really* think I was good?"

"You were better than good. You were fantastic!"

Deb spent the night, and the next morning I found her and Jess in the living room, doing yoga. I left the room for a few moments to put some breakfast on the table, and when I returned they were both standing on their heads against the wall.

"Look at me, Mommy!" Jessica squealed.

"I'm looking," I said. "You look different."

"That's because I'm upside down!"

Deb and Jessica became closer with each visit, and Deb never tired of telling my daughter wonderful things about me. "Your mother is a great surgeon and an amazing woman, Jessica—did you know that?"

"You told me already," Jessica would say.

"Well, I'm telling you again so you won't forget."

And of course there was always shopping, which was risky for anyone with a limited income and bills to pay.

"I approach shopping from a unique point of view," Deb explained. "It's probably dangerous for someone without ovarian cancer to go shopping with me."

She was right. She didn't expect to be around long enough to have to worry about money, and her attitude was contagious. I found myself thinking, *Well, she's right! We never know what's going to happen to us, so we might as well enjoy life as fully as we can.* I ended up doing some serious financial damage, but I must say I enjoyed myself in the process, and I always stopped short of *total* fiscal irresponsibility.

One morning, Deb asked me why I had gone into gynecologic oncology since I could just as easily have opted for obstetrics. I told her that it was primarily because of the intensity of the relationships with my patients. Before I had committed to the field, I had thought about obstetrics and gynecology, but I found the risk of potential litigation very frustrating. I never felt like I was on the same team as the patient and her baby, so I seemed to be practicing defensive medicine.

In cancer care, on the other hand, the good and the bad players are obvious. The patient is good, and, in many cases, innocent, and the cancer is bad. The doctor and the drugs are part of the armamentarium. I saw my patients as victims, as the underdogs in need of help.

"I'm not sure I like your interpretation of ovarian cancer patients as 'victims,'" Deb said.

"I'm using the term broadly," I said, upset at having offended her.

"I still don't like it," she said.

I understood. Deb didn't want to feel like a victim. She wanted to feel that she was in control, and that she could fight this Goddamn thing—and fight it successfully.

It was only later, when she watched her close friend Fran Lantz succumb to ovarian cancer, that Deb wavered. In a sense, she was looking at her own future, and she didn't like it. Fran was taking nourishment intravenously, and, as Deb put it, she had become a living skeleton.

"That's not the way I'm going to go," Deb told me. "I want a stash of morphine and enough potassium to stop my heart, and I'll leave on my own terms. I will lie in a hammock and play Mozart loudly enough to wake the neighbors. That's what I'm going to do. I'm going to be in control."

For the first three years of her cancer drama, my friend Fran Lantz never took antinausea drugs at home. The ones that were given to her before the infusion of chemotherapy seemed to suffice. Alternatively, I have spent much of my time close to nausea.

Elaine Scarry wrote The Body in Pain. *In it, she is looking at pain generated from human torture. She makes an interesting argument that finally some pain is beyond our ability to describe or to voice. It is simply a shriek of sorts or a cry of desperation. When I would see my physicians at M. D. Anderson, there was generally a list of symptoms I would fill out in advance of seeing the doctor. For the first five years of my cancer experience, reading the form that asked me to describe my pain on a scale from one to ten didn't make sense to me. Now that I am more symptomatic and have had* the morphine-at-home experience, I understand the questions. But for much of my treatment I looked for a different way to express what I was feeling. Was it the Buddhist dukkha? Was I suffering, experiencing an unsatisfactoriness in the present that was made more palpable when I remembered how I had felt before cancer became my dharma? Was I feeling "punk," as my grandmother used to say? Was it the baldness and perpetually being cold that bothered me? Nausea is centered in the tummy, but it changes the way you see and the way you walk, if you are walking at all.

I developed a game when I first went to M. D. Anderson, and I continued to play it. M. D. Anderson represents a modern pilgrimage site. It is a place where people come to be given a second opinion or a second chance at life. M. D. Anderson's tag advertising line—Making Cancer History—is both a statement of fact and a promise of hope for its patients. For many people, M. D. Anderson puts cancer in their past; for others, it extends the time they have in the present. A diagnosis of cancer doesn't change the way you look. It's the treatment that causes you to be bald or thin or just puny. But to be fair, the disease will sooner or later do it to you too. People who come to M. D. Anderson generally don't come alone. Spouses, sisters, brothers, parents, and kids of all sizes make the trip with the patient.

That was the game. I would try to identify the patient when I would see a group that possessed a certain family resemblance coming toward me in the maze of hallways that connect the various departments at the clinic. In some cases, it was obvious: the mask, the plastic gloves, the IV pole or portable hydration pack, and the plastic tubing that disappeared into the shirt that buttoned or zipped up the front. (No pullover shirts for cancer patients. It is too difficult for the nurses to get to the catheter that is placed in the chest. Alternatively, a patient can have a net sleeve that keeps an access site available on the arm.) However, early on, before treatment starts, these roving bands of similar looking people, all ambulatory, all eating well at the clinic's various restaurants and cafeterias, looked as though they could be on vacation. Of course, they were not. Strange to say it, but everyone I met in cancer care was civil and invariably kind. All were brave and most were full of courtesy. Two examples will illustrate my point:

Early on in my care, before I had the recurrence that required BMT, I met a perfectly beautiful African-American woman while we were in the "pen," where people wait for a CT scan. I had noticed her in the waiting room, in part because she looked so healthy. We were both dressed in hospital blue and waiting for the IV nurse to insert the plug to enable the technician to deliver the iodine contrast that makes for a more readable scan. As I learned in the course of our conversation, she was a mother of grown daughters (though she hardly looked it), and had been diagnosed with Stage IV pancreatic cancer some nine months previously. Both of us knew that she should be dead by now. It was a miracle, and it was her extraordinary Christian faith and the act of a loving God that was keeping her well, singing, and in the world. Quite apart from her religious conviction, I liked her very much. We exchanged phone numbers, and I did call her once. In truth, I was afraid to call her again. I did not want to hear how it had gone, since in either case, for me, it would be bad news. If she was well—and I keenly wished this for her—it would reflect the *power of prayer and remind me that I was not a person of this sort of faith. If she was ill or, God forbid, dead, then it was just another case of the triumph of cancer's invincible power.*

My second example is in some ways both less personal for me and more instructive. Again, in the holding pen of the CT scan department, I found myself sitting next to a lovely young woman, painfully thin, from southern India. She told me that she had just given birth to her second child and that she was a nurse at another hospital in Houston. Thin, so thin, she told me that she had been diagnosed with esophageal cancer, and that she was about to begin a round of chemotherapy that would presumably shrink the tumor sufficiently so that it could then be removed surgically. I assumed she was a Hindu, having come to Houston just three years previously. But when the IV nurse came to her and began to insert the needle into her arm, the young mother murmured quietly, "Thank you, Jesus. Thank you, Jesus."

I understood only too well what Deb was referring to. This is one of life's inexplicable mysteries. I see patients of great intrinsic faith and I think, *I want what they have.* The irony is that many of my patients are poor and have little else. These are the women I talked about earlier, the "underserved," the "indigent." They are often women who have suffered countless indignities in their lives, but as the end draws near a great many of them seem to find peace of mind. For them, destiny is a given—unalterable and beyond control. Faith seems to have played a huge role in their lives, and in talking to them I sometimes get the impression that they don't believe that any changes here on earth will affect the final outcome. I am always surprised—and somewhat honored, too—when a patient looks up at me, innocent and full of trust, and says, "Whatever you say, doctor. Just do what you think is best."

Most of those patients are at the county hospital. Most of my patients at M. D. Anderson, the academic hospital, may or may not have that level of faith in God, but most of them believe that they have some control over their own destinies— and, as a result, over the types of treatment they receive. If I were a patient, I would be in this latter camp. My parents taught me to believe that I controlled my future, and I still believe it—even to the point of self-delusion. Now, on a daily basis, I was being asked to take control over other people's futures, and it made me think about the tenuousness of all our lives, including my own.

"Lois," one of my mentors used to say, "no guts, no glory."

It took a while for me to realize that he was talking about this very subject: the power that a trusting patient places in the hands of his or her doctor. While the patient slept, I was being trusted to make the right strategic decisions for her. We were going to battle, and I was the general, running the show.

It also took me a while to realize that it was my responsibility, as the doctor-general, to keep my patient informed about all the risks that she'd be facing. I am not sure all doctors would agree with me, but this is the way I practice medicine. I can only do battle—and it *is* battle—by being completely honest with my patients. And I refuse to abandon them when things don't go as planned. I will remain by their side even when the battle is lost.

There is always hope, of course. Hope makes it possible to undergo the pain of surgery and the side effects of chemotherapy. Hope makes a believer of both the patient and the doctor, makes them think that *this* is the rare patient who will survive. But when the cancer returns—when, as Deb says, "one leaves the Remission Society"—the battle metaphor no longer works. We can continue to manage the pain, the nausea, the visible tumors, the body parts that have already succumbed, but at that point there really is no hope, at that point there is nothing left to fight for.

I generally get to that place before the patient does, because this is what I do every day, this is my profession, but I invariably look for a way out. *Have I done something wrong? Have I forgotten anything? Is there still a possibility? What have I missed?*

Then, finally, we have The Talk, and the patient and I try to find peace of mind together.

In July 2003, Jessica and I made our second trip to California. Deb and Giles had moved to the beach house in Ventura, determined to grab life by the horns, and were both happier for it. The home was truly a paradise. They went to sleep to the sound of the waves and woke to the peaceful calm of the sea, literally at their doorstep. I remember sitting with my daughter on the gigantic rocks in front of their house, reading and looking at the waves, and feeling as relaxed as I'd ever felt. I also remember doing yoga next to Deb, on the deck, with the ocean breezes washing over us.

"I think a number of things are contributing to your longevity," I told her one night. "The yoga, the massages, your painting, the way you laugh, and, of course, this magical place."

"What about the inordinate amounts of broccoli I eat?" she asked, laughing her big laugh.

"That, too," I said.

"It's probably the headstands, though. I'm suffocating the tumors by denying them oxygen."

When Deb was resting, Jessica and I went for walks on the beach, poking around tide pools filled with starfish and sea anemones. We also bonded over one of my favorite book collections, Lemony Snicket's *A Series of Unfortunate Events*. I liked the books because they were well written, but mostly I liked them because they steered clear of happy, fairy-tale endings.

It was during this trip that I first met Deb's son, Adam, now in his thirties, who had come into Deb's life though Giles's previous marriage, and whom Deb regarded as her own. This had not occurred overnight, but Deb took great pride in that Adam regarded her as "Mom," especially since he had had his share of problems earlier in life. A dyslexic kid with three parents holding Ph.D.s, it had taken Adam a long time to gain academic traction after high school. Deb still saw him for what he was, however—an exceptionally bright kid with a real talent for science, but not much patience for academia. While he was still in college, at the University of California, Santa Barbara, he went to work for a computer company and became a systems analyst, and he remains with the same company to this day—a valued and respected employee. By the time Deb was diagnosed, Adam was fully in control of his life, and firmly back in the fold. He was at the house for dinner at least once a week, and after the family moved to the beach he was there every weekend, just to "hang out," as he told Deb. I found him to be very good company, and also supremely helpful. Adam was forever shopping, cooking, running errands, and solving computer problems, and he always did it with a smile.

During this visit, one other thing I noticed was the way Deb and Giles said goodbye, which was very different from the habits of my own family. Their goodbyes were short and sweet, unlike the emotional and painfully drawn out goodbyes of my childhood and adolescence. Interestingly, in my family, we had never had any real tragedy, so these emotional partings made little sense. We seemed to live with the unreasonable fear that each goodbye could be the last. For Deb and Giles, the shared time is what counts, not the parting moments. When they say goodbye, it's with the knowledge that they'll be seeing each other again.

By this time, I felt so close to Deb that I could talk to her about absolutely anything. One of my more pervasive worries was about my ex-husband Ross's fiancée, and the role she was soon to play in Jessica's life as Ross's wife—in particular

over the issue of religious faith. Deb was the perfect person
with whom to discuss this. She knew my ex-husband was an
agnostic, but his new wife was a Baptist, and Jessica had been
coming home recently with all sorts of questions about the
nature of good and evil.

"I don't know if she should be talking to Jessica about
good and evil," I complained to Deb. "Wouldn't that be like
buying a dog for the other person's house?"

"In effect, yes—precisely."

Jessica, who was eight then, had come home one day
asking, "Who is our Savior?" So I read to her from *What is
God?*, a book by Etan Boritzer that I'd bought shortly after she
was born. The book looks at the major religions of the world,
and at the teachers and prophets representing them—Jesus,
Moses, Mohammed, and Buddha. It also discusses the Bible,
the Torah, the Koran, the Sutras, and the Vedas, and explains
that prayer is universal—that all of us are simply trying to
connect with God.

"So what *is* God?" she asked.

"Everyone asks what God is," I said, "but nobody knows.
Every religion is different, and every religion has its own
ideas, but one idea isn't better than any other idea."

"What is God to you?" she asked.

"It's hard to put into words, but in this book, the author
says that, to him, God is when he closes his eyes and breathes
in and out, and that this breathing makes him feel connected
to other people. And when he hears thunder, he feels that that
is the power of God. And that is also what I believe."

When I told Deb what I'd told my daughter, she thought that it was as valid a description as any. She wasn't a fan of organized religion—she thought organized religion tended to be exclusionary, and she couldn't condone that—but she still liked to think of herself as a Jew. "I'm not a practicing Jew, but I'm a Jew, and it's part of my identity," she said. "But I don't look at other people and think, 'Oh, she's a non-Jew.'"

It was interesting, because Abby had a friend at the time who was very religious. Deb often referred to him as the Preacher, although not in a mean-spirited way. "I worry that Abby's going to get converted," she said, only half-joking.

"To what?"

"I don't know," she said, laughing. "That's partly what worries me."

When Jessica and I returned to Houston, Nuri and I started getting closer than ever, and I began to feel cautiously optimistic about our future. He had patience and an emotional intelligence that was good for both my daughter and me. I was particularly impressed by his deep-seated ability to enjoy the moment. He worried very little about the future, knowing already that it was uncertain and that no amount of worrying would change anything. He began trying to teach me to enjoy every moment of every day, and I started getting better at it, but I am still learning.

Meanwhile, I was dealing with the usual trials and tribulations of every divorced parent.

"I don't have to go to bed at Daddy's house till nine!"

"Well, this is not Daddy's house, and the rules are different here."

"I like the rules better there."

"Then you can enjoy them when you're over there."

Sometimes, when Jessica got angry about some trifle or other, she'd threaten to call her father, and one day I finally sat her down and tried to give her the tools to deal with her frustration. "Every parent has his or her own style, and you're going to have to get used to it," I said. "When you have a problem at this house, let's deal with it at this house."

I hated arguing with her, and I felt guilty when I disciplined her, partly because I didn't feel I was spending enough time just being a mother. But then I realized that she was turning into a really neat kid, and that the parenting mistakes I'd made didn't seem to have done any irreparable damage.

One night, as I was thinking about my parenting skills, or lack of them, Deb reached me on the phone. "How would you like to go to Paris with me?" she asked.

"Paris?"

"I'm going with a group of people from the university, but you and I can share a room. I know we'll have a great time together."

I really didn't know what to do. I had never traveled much and wasn't a fan of flying, and I felt terribly guilty about leaving Jessica behind with her father and his fiancée. It wasn't really them, though—they were perfectly decent people. It was mostly me.

"I can't leave Jessie alone for ten whole days," I told Deb, trying to focus on the legitimate part of my hesitation. "She'll miss me too much."

"Or you her," she said.

"Okay," I replied. "That, too."

"I think you'll both survive," Deb said. "You don't have to decide this very moment, but at least think about it."

On December 21, Deb, growing impatient, wrote in an e-mail:

> Lois, dear—look at the kid. You are a great mother. But if you want I will join in your pity-party all the way to Paris. . . . I am feeling quite well and I don't have much hair, but plenty of hats.

Finally, she agreed to meet me in Houston so that we could fly to Paris together.

On my way to the airport, I kept asking myself, *What are you afraid of? Deb has the cancer. Certainly she should be more scared!* But a moment later, I'd flip this around: *Why should Deb be scared? She has cancer. She has nothing to lose if the plane crashes!*

When we rendezvoused at the airport, Deb greeted me with her usual big laugh and a friendly hug, but she could see I was in horrible distress.

"Open your mouth," she said.

I did as I was told, and she popped an Ativan under my tongue. Without it, I don't think I would have boarded the plane.

On the flight over, under the influence of my little tranquilizer, I told Deb that I had been asked to write a review on spirituality and gynecologic oncology for an international journal, and that I'd been thinking about the topic for so long that I thought there was a book in it. "Would you be interested in writing it with me?" I asked.

"Absolutely," she said, visibly delighted. "Both of us certainly have a lot to say on the subject."

"We sure do," I agreed.

Paris was absolutely wonderful. We were both completely free and felt it. We shopped, we walked, we people-watched, and we talked. I remember one particularly fun moment when we stopped at a wig shop, a significant place for a cancer patient. We each tried on our share of wigs, laughing at our reflections in the store mirror. Deb was completely bald by this time, but she left without a wig. "I have nothing to hide," she said.

One morning, we walked all the way to the top of the Eiffel Tower, which was hard on her.

"If Giles were here, would he let you do this?"

"Of course not!" she said. "That's why I came with you!"

"I'm really glad you talked me into coming."

She turned to me and smiled. "You know, Lois, I know we've talked about this before, but it really does make it much easier—the fact that you've only ever known me as a cancer patient. You accept me for who I am. You don't expect me to be the person I was before I got sick."

The next day, we went to a Turkish bathhouse. We lay naked on heated marble slabs and women scrubbed us down with loofahs. Given the potential for infection, this went against my better judgment as a doctor, but we were having too good a time to worry about such things.

In the mornings, before Deb was awake, I would go jogging through the streets and along the Seine, past bridges of ancient stone. When I returned Deb would be waiting for me in the breakfast room, sipping tea. Every day was a new adventure. The Picasso museum. The Champs-Élysées. The cobbled streets of the Left Bank.

One day, we had lunch at a little café next to the Louvre. Both of us were very excited. We had been talking about the book we hoped to write, and we decided that, at heart, it needed to be about our unusual friendship: She, a professor of religion, struggling with cancer, and me, her doctor, trying to make sense of this whole notion of mortality, in my patients, myself, and, most pointedly, in my new friend.

"This is what people in my field would call a 'crisis of meaning,'" Deb said.

Ironically, it was our mutual interest in spirituality, and in the art of dying specifically, that had brought us to this place. Our first journal article had dealt with this very topic. The book would be a more detailed exploration of much the same, but the approach needed to be more human, less clinical.

Deb pulled out a notebook and made a few notes as we talked, and I read over her shoulder. "You write like an academic college professor," I said, laughing.

"Ya *think*?" she shot at me.

"Yes. I think."

"Well, I *am* an academic college professor!"

"I was trained to write in short, clear sentences," I told her archly.

"Really?" she said, laughing. "From what I've seen, you write like a doctor."

"What, messy and illegible?" I said, laughing. "We're going to have to find a happy medium."

"Maybe we can write in both of our voices. I'll write my academic part and you'll write your doctor part and we'll make it work."

"That's not a bad idea," I said.

At that point, I noticed a woman at a nearby table, eating alone but watching us—watching us laughing and ribbing each other and having fun. Not long after, she paid her bill, and on her way out she stopped by our table.

"Excuse me," she said in English heavily accented by French. "I have been watching you, and I must say . . ." She turned to look at Deb now. "There's a powerful light coming from inside of you!"

"Really!" Deb said, laughing. "It's very kind of you to say so. Thank you."

It was true. The positive energy in Deb was unbelievable. She could light up a whole room. She lit up that entire Parisian café!

Two nights later, Deb took me out for a birthday dinner at Le Grand Colbert. I was thirty-seven. "I feel old," I said.

"Old? I've just passed fifty."

The fact that she had almost *not* made it to fifty was left unsaid.

"You know," she continued, "I don't view cancer as a gift, but if it wasn't for the cancer we never would have met."

"We need to put that in the book," I said quietly.

"Yes, we do," she said.

I returned from Paris rejuvenated, and not long after, in January 2004, Deb sent me a rough draft of the introduction to our proposed book, which said, in part:

> Recently, there has been a great deal of interest among oncologists and other medical personnel about the connection between what researchers have called "a patient's spirituality" and the progress of his or her disease. The literature has become legion and it runs from patients' peculiar medical autobiographies to clinical research on the ostensible interrelationship between what we call "health" and the cancer experience. . . .
>
> Oncologists too are in a peculiar position, some might say a peculiarly *metaphysical* position. Physicians have access to individuals who are *in extremis*, individuals who are confronting "the distinguished thing" as Henry James called it. For oncologists, death is part of the arc of their work with patients. And, not surprisingly, physicians and nurses report that they are both fascinated and frightened by the tremendous mystery that death presents to their patients, and for them as observers. Virtually all oncologists know a "good death" when they see one. They also know "bad

ones," ones that invoke a sense of meaninglessness for the patient and the patient's family. . . .

This is a book that brings theory and practice together. It is a book about the peculiar vocabularies that both patients and oncologists use to describe their life and times in the Kingdom of the Ill. It is also about the ways in which patients and physicians meet each other, come to construct a mutual world of meanings that inform their respective experiences in the world of oncological medicine.

After I looked at it, and discussed it with Deb, we were simultaneously excited and frustrated. We knew there was a book in there, but we didn't know exactly what it was. Then Deb discussed it with Giles, and he understood it immediately.

"It is a book about two women from two completely different worlds, trying to come to grips with the mystery of mortality," he said.

Later, when I thought about how eloquently he'd summed it up, I realized something else about the book: For me, it was an intellectual and emotional exercise. For Deb, it was real; it was what was left.

7

SPIRITUALITY AND CANCER

In March 2004, Nuri took Jessica and me to Dubai to meet his brother and his family. My mother was very concerned. "What do I do if you get kidnapped?"

"You think Nuri is going to kidnap me?!"

"Not Nuri. Anybody. You're Jewish, remember? And it's an Arab country."

"Mom, I'm not going to get abducted or held for ransom. This is not a TV movie." Suddenly, after one overseas trip to Paris, I had become a fearless traveler.

That said, the adventure began the moment we arrived with the airline losing our luggage. We had to borrow clothes from Nuri's family for our first foray into the city, where I was in for another surprise: Dubai was surprisingly modern, with gleaming high-rises everywhere, blotting out the sky. The next day, however, after a thirty-minute drive north, we found ourselves in an area where women covered themselves in public, and this felt a lot closer to what I'd seen in *National Geographic*.

We visited various markets, including one in Sharjah, a neighboring emirate. We were surrounded by colors and sounds and scents that were uniquely foreign. Nuri and I bought a wonderful rug and some Afghani jewelry, mostly lapis lazuli. We also explored the desert, where we rode a camel and learned to sand-surf, which was the highlight of the trip for Jessica.

While we were there, Deb e-mailed to say that she had been invited to lecture at Bogazici University, where Nuri had actually attended school for a year, in Bebek, near Istanbul, Turkey. This was the second time they had asked her to go, and she had previously been too sick to consider it, but she really wanted to do it this time. She told me she had been talking to the team at M. D. Anderson about putting her on a special regimen to prepare her for the trip. She needed eight full weeks without chemotherapy, which was doable but still worrisome. "They're all so concerned," Deb told me. "But they don't seem to understand: I have decided that I'm going to spend whatever time I have left the way I want to spend it. I need everyone to be on my side."

I was also worried for other reasons. During Deb's previous visit, there had been bombings in Istanbul and Ankara to protest the North Atlantic Treaty Organization. I wanted to say something about this, but I didn't want to sound like a mother.

By late April, Deb was deep into her new medical regimen, getting ready for her trip to Turkey and feeling fairly stable, so I flew out to Santa Barbara for a long weekend to work on our book. We worked on the deck overlooking the ocean, and at night I would fall asleep to the crash and roar of the surf. It was heavenly.

In the morning, Deb and I would go back to work, but by noon we had made our way into Santa Barbara, to shop and spend money I didn't have. In the afternoon, we would work a little more, and in the evenings Giles would come home and make martinis.

One night we read parts of the book aloud to him, taking turns, and he was hugely enthusiastic. I was excited, too. Listening to Deb read from the sections she'd written, and hearing my own very different voice, made me think we had really hit on something.

On my last afternoon there, I went outside and found Deb lying in the hammock in the sun. She had just finished reading *Tuesdays with Morrie*, the huge bestseller by Mitch Albom, about his weekly visits to a dying friend. "We can do better than this," she said.

I returned to Houston—to Jessica, to Nuri, and to the long hours at the hospital—and in June, Deb left for Turkey. One of her very first lectures, not surprisingly, was about illness and renewal—about our touchstone issue of the intersection of cancer care, women's experiences, and quality-of-life issues.

The trip to Turkey was only partly academic. Deb and Giles had decided to follow it up with a cruise in the Aegean with friends, and they were going to take Abby with them. Giles had a fairly serious motorcycle accident just before their departure, however, and Abby fell down the stairs and hurt herself the week before. It was touch and go if everyone would actually make it, but they did—Abby just off crutches and Giles now back on them for a while.

Giles shared some of the e-mails he received from Deb in the weeks before he and Abby flew out to meet her:

I teach tomorrow and need to think about how all this will go. Teaching feminism here [in Turkey] is a very different business than doing it in California!

Oh Giles, I've been reading Carolyn Heilbrun on marriage and get to talk about it tomorrow [in class]. Do I miss talking to you about virtually anything! A Greek salad tonight, here in the apartment, and then I finished reading Shirley Lim's autobio.

I had a drink at the Bebek Hotel . . . on the terrace overlooking the Bosphorus. Giles, you are going to love it here!

The traffic in Istanbul is horrific and getting around, apart from the feet, is a feat. I am home tonight reading up on Madness and Confinement and will go to bed early. It is really a good idea. I have a very full day tomorrow. Teaching, office hours, and then a faculty event in the evening. It is a party at a downtown hotel to celebrate the appointment of a new rector to the university. She is a very good-looking and very elegant mathematician. I met her for the first time last week on the dance floor. A woman mathematician and wow—can she dance!

I am now about to make some dinner—it's 7:30 here— and get to bed early. I like to get up around 6 and get myself ready [for class]. The boats out the window are wonderful. It is our favorite time of day, martini time, and the light is just right and the colors of the boats—white, red, blue, and more—are lovely against the blue of the Bosphorus. More later and much much love, me

Dearest, we are coming up on our anniversary and I am growing lonely at the distance that is between us. Imagine the life that we have created for ourselves.

Sweet Love, I imagine that you are in class right now and I am about to go off to bed, read Zora Neale Hurston's autobiography, and then have a really long sleep. It has been a long and yet really wonderful week and I am tired and I'm thinking about all that you have done this week. Sorting out the money for our blue [Aegean] voyage, the global studies meetings, not to mention teaching two classes each day and thinking about Abby. . . . What an adventure I have had with you, Mr. Gunn, and am I a lucky girl! Love you to pieces, me

I am thrilled that the two of you are coming. Bring a hat—it is hot in the sun—and your shorts and some wash pants and a bathing suit. Also shoes to walk in.

Tomorrow I don't teach but hope to get my work done for the week. I will have a good number of papers to begin grading on Monday. I am taking the bus now and feel somewhat like a local.

I am looking forward to your arrival more than I can say. What I am afraid of is that I will just talk once you arrive. I have been strangely silent and alone these last weeks and I will try to remember that others—ie, you and Abby—also have items on your mind.

How about [bringing me] a New Yorker or the NY Review of Books? I did the archeological museums on Sunday and the big Mosque on the hill, which can mean that you don't have to. We can talk about it. Being in the town is hot, and the standing in museums hard on the feet. And yet, one sees [everything] up close—close enough to touch.

Love you. Me

. . .

Deb and Abby also communicated frequently via e-mail, and Abby was kind enough to share some of them. These were sent in June and July of 2004:

It was really wonderful to hear your voice this morning. It is now about 9 and I am about to get ready to go to school. It is raining here in Istanbul and lots of thunder. I am reading just about anything I want to and move about this lovely apartment like an aging college student, or what I remember about my own graduate life before I married Giles. . . . Does your mother love you? Bunches and bunches and thank you for your letter. Be safe and enjoy and more love and kisses, Mommeles

My life is really quite tame. Talks with [my friend] Chantal, walks by the Bosphorus, yoga, reading, teaching, more reading, listening to music, conversation with some wonderful Turkish women academics, and, finally, a perfectly splendid evening at the Topkapi Palace, listening to baroque music. This does sound like an old woman writing, but I am really having a great time. . . . When you have time, write me a note. I am very tickled that you and Dad are coming to Istanbul. I will know my way around by then and will have tales to tell and places to go. I love you kid, your momma xxxooo

Ablet, I understand that you are not feeling well, swollen glands et al. Please child take care of yourself and drink lots of water and take vitamin C. . . . Love you so much and can't wait to show you Istanbul. The Mominator

I have been meaning to tell you about the cats in Istanbul. They are everywhere and no one touches them, but sometimes people feed them. If you don't feed them they can jump up and attack. Haven't seen a fat one yet. Buddy would run the place, and Maxx would never have survived here. What this indicates about the cultural lives of the Turks I cannot say. . . . Feel better sweet girl and I wish I could make you a cup of honey with lemon juice, your momma

Hello Abby dear . . . and there is some irony here that I am writing to you from Istanbul to tell you to CLEAN UP YOUR ROOM. Do things ever change?

The wonderful thing, Abby dear, is that I am proud of you with or without a messy room. I am spending a good deal of my time on my class. The days are quiet and yoga is good and it is a surprisingly restful and restorative place. I teach today and so I am off to shower and put on the face. You remember the face?—the one with the big reddish lips and no eyebrows. More later and much love, Mommeles

I think my class is going well, but I will know later when I read their evaluations. I am coming up to speed on American slavery and women's autobiography and it is grim—a really grim business. A kind of sexual terrorism overlaid the lives of slave women. They were often chosen by white owners as concubines and then the children from these unions were often sold away from their moms. Oy.

I'm back to class for office hours and then to a film noir, "Kiss me Deadly." Can you imagine? I get to see some of my favorite 40s films here! Get your bathing suit ready and bring a hat, not a big one, but one of those little porkpie jobs. Do you know what I mean?

My sweetest Ablet, I am so sorry that you are on crutches and that the foot—or is it the ankle—is hurt? I really want you to come to Turkey. I had a night dancing to gypsy music on the streets of Istanbul. Can you believe this, after eating salad and fish? My idea of a good time, how about yours?

Did I tell you that I tried to sell encyclopedias door to door in my youth and that I was not any good at it?

Dearest Ablet, When I wrote "Be here now," I was quoting both the Dalai Lama and Ram Dass, aka

Richard Alpert, a former sidekick of Timothy Leary. It is not so much about "place" as "time." Being in the present helps one not to worry about the future and not to be bitter about the past.

I have been reading about this new psychotherapy in the Herald Tribune, called "dialectial behavioral therapy," which is used with suicidal patients and people with eating disorders. It runs something like this: When a patient tells the therapist that he or she wants to commit suicide, the therapist says "Why not?" and "Why not now?" and it goes from there. Presumably the patient then comes to a point where he or she says they want to live and then the issue is: It is just an emotional storm and it will pass and you don't have to act on your feelings. Really rather Buddhist, I think. One becomes an observer in one's own drama. The Buddhist term would be to be "mindful."

Living alone like this, I am watching much of life and participating in it, too. More on this later and I too am looking forward to an Abby snuggle, big time. Keep the foot up and use a cane. Think of yourself as an Oscar Wilde redux.

After the Aegean cruise, which Deb described to me in superlatives—*amazing, fantastic, unforgettable*—the family returned to Santa Barbara, and Deb left a little note on Giles's desk, simply to let him know how much she appreciated him:

Giles dear

I went to Europe as a recovering sick person—full of fear about my stamina, my health, + my resources. . . .

. . . and I've come home to you well and full of life's vital power.

What a gift you have given me!

How is it that you're so smart?

I'm so glad to be home w/ you.

Much love from me

Deb

On August 16, 2004, Nuri's father died, and Nuri returned to Amman to help arrange the funeral. His father had been a doctor in the Jordanian army, and he was buried with full military honors. Nuri e-mailed to say that people kept stopping him to tell him stories about his father, all of whom described him in glowing terms. Nuri was very moved, especially since his father had been suffering from Alzheimer's for the past decade and had already been "missing" for many years.

I did not accompany Nuri to Amman because I didn't want to meet his mother under those circumstances. He e-mailed every day, however, and sent text messages, and he told me that he took long walks through the city every day to deal with his sadness.

I thought back to the weeks preceding Nuri's father's death, when his mother called to say that he had developed pneumonia and was on a ventilator. I had gone into Doctor-Mode and tried to talk to Nuri about what he could expect, medically speaking, but he didn't want to talk about it. As he explained it, in his culture one accepts these things as God's will. They even have an expression for it: *Enshallah*.

My relationship with Nuri continued to deepen and enrich me in unexpected ways. Nuri was teaching me to enjoy the present—to be in the *now*, as Deb had put it—and I was getting the hang of it, albeit in tiny increments. Nuri would see joy in little, everyday things: hanging out with Jessica and me. Talking on the phone to his family. Cooking. Listening to music. Taking long, leisurely, aimless walks around the neighborhood. He was teaching me, by example, to savor each moment.

"When you come home, I want you to forget everything that happened at the hospital today," he would say. "You are here. With your family. This is all that matters."

He was never impatient. There was never an angry word from him. Never a negative comment. Never any criticism.

Sometimes, just before we would sit down to dinner, he would reach for my hand, hold it for a second, and look at me. Just for a second, maybe two. It felt almost like a form of prayer. It was his way of giving thanks, and it filled me with gratitude, too—for my life, for my daughter, for Nuri. "Whatever happens," he once told me, "you need to remember that you can get through it, and that everything always works out."

Not long after Nuri returned to Houston, Deb called to tell me that Giles had been invited to deliver a series of lectures in Turkey, and that she had loved the land so much that she intended to return with him. She asked if Nuri and I would join them. "You'll love it," she said. "It is a wonderful country. I need you to come."

I said I'd think about it—and I did—but I didn't see how I could get away. Then I changed the subject. "I've been asked to speak at an ovarian cancer conference in December, which is going to be hosted by M. D. Anderson. I already have a title for my lecture: 'Spirituality and Ovarian Cancer: How, Why, When?' Would you be interested in lecturing with me and flying to Houston in December for the presentation?"

"Absolutely!" Deb said.

"We also have to work on the book," I said.

"Shit, yes, Lois!" she said. "We need to get moving."

Deb and Giles were going to be leaving for Turkey in October, and in the preceding weeks Deb kept asking me to join them, and to bring Nuri. I kept waffling. I had work, of course, but I was more worried about leaving Jessica behind. At one point I asked Jess if she would be upset if Nuri and I went on a short vacation, and she looked at me like an exasperated teenager. "Mom! Why would I be upset?"

I remembered thinking, *Couldn't you at least* pretend *that you'll miss me a little?*

The following day I found a cheap flight and told Nuri

about it. He didn't think he could get away, but he urged me to go ahead and book it, and I did.

A week later, on October 5, 2004, I e-mailed Deb with the news:

Subject: The hour is drawing near

Deb, I am excited to say that Nuri has just informed me that he is working very hard in order to go with us. He has bought tickets on the same flight as me and is coming! I am very glad, although I informed him that I need "Deb time" to talk and he would have to wander! Hopefully this won't be a problem with the reservations in the hotel. Should I change anything? This is very exciting!!!

She replied in short order:

Lois dear, it looks like we are really going—and yes, Giles tells me that Asli is making reservations for you and for us at the Bebek Hotel for the days you are with us apart from our time at the Hotel Empress Zoe. The Bebek is wonderful and all of us will be well taken care of there.

What more can I tell you? I am finishing up a report for the Honors Committee and then turning my attention to our paper and our project. Don't worry about clothes, I will take you to Figan—do you need a suit or something for evening balls? More later and much love, Deb

. . .

Turkey was as terrific as Paris, and more exotic. When we arrived at the hotel, after a long, overnight flight, Deb and Giles were already out on the town, but there was a beautiful breakfast buffet laid out in the lobby—meats, olives, various cheeses—and we loaded our plates and carried them into the quaint courtyard. We sat at a small iron table, and not half an hour later I heard a loud, familiar laugh. We looked up to see Deb and Giles moving toward us, framed against the stone archway. It felt like a dream. We hugged and kissed and they joined us for breakfast, and then the four of us went off to explore the city—the mosques, the secret gardens tucked behind ancient walls, the slow-moving ferries.

I remember stepping onto my hotel balcony late that afternoon, as the prayers were being broadcast, ringing out across the city, and lifting my camera to get a picture of the dwindling light. I found Deb on the neighboring balcony, with her own camera, and we laughed and took pictures of each other.

"I'm so happy you talked me into coming," I told her the next day. We were walking arm in arm through one of the famous markets, imitating the local women. Giles and Nuri were behind us, trailing, and Nuri was constantly getting lost.

"Where is your man disappearing to all the time?" Deb asked jokingly. "Is he like this at home?"

We walked everywhere together, and ate constantly. Deb had some of her appetite back, but she was noticeably less energetic than she'd been in Paris. She never lost her enthusiasm, though. We went to cafés, played backgammon with the locals, drank exotic teas, and, yes, worked on the book.

It was Ramadan while we were there, a time of fasting, and at sunset we would see veiled women lining up with their families, getting ready to eat after a full day without food or drink. It made me feel a little guilty: My belly was always full of hummus, lamb, fish, and all manner of fancy desserts.

From time to time, Deb and I actually ventured out on our own, to see the sights and to shop. I bought a lot of turquoise, which was impossible to resist at those prices, and Deb—well, Deb bought *everything*. Earrings. Hats. Scarves splashed with bold colors. Spices.

One day, I went off on my own to visit several hospitals— something I had arranged through M. D. Anderson—and it was late by the time I returned to the Bebek Hotel. I was on the ferry, alone, and as the only Westerner I stood out. I felt simultaneously adventurous and nervous.

But when I walked into my hotel room, the whole world suddenly changed. There were dozens of burning candles everywhere, and the floor was covered with flower petals, and Nuri was waiting for me on bended knee. He asked me to marry him, and I took a deep breath—inhaling the scent of the flowers—and accepted before he could change his mind.

When we returned home, just as we were beginning to plan our wedding, Deb took a sudden and unexpected turn for the worse. One of her California doctors found a suspicious nodule on her lung, and the most likely explanation was that the cancer had returned, manifesting itself in a new location. I hoped it might be something else. "It could be tuberculosis," I told Deb. "You might have picked it up in Turkey."

"Is that really possible?"

"Possible," I said, then, almost against my will: "But not likely."

At the urging of Dr. Bouquet, Deb made arrangements to fly to Houston for a biopsy, and I braced myself for the worst. Patients with ovarian cancer usually have Stage III disease at diagnosis. It truly is the silent killer, sneaking up on women with very subtle symptoms. I often tell my students that the symptoms are similar to the ones you might have after gorging yourself at a Mexican restaurant. Bloating; burping; sudden, unexplained exhaustion—discomforts you can live with for three or four months before you even consider checking it out. At that point, most women will see a gastrointestinal special ist, and might even undergo an endoscopy or a colonoscopy, but nothing is found. As a result, a lot of damage has already been done by the time the cancer is detected.

Often, the cancer cells have had time to implant themselves on the bowel walls and on the lining of the abdomen, and even to produce fluids (ascites). When this occurs, a woman can find, over a period of weeks, her abdomen swelling very quickly—frighteningly so. This is usually the point when a CT is ordered and the tumor is discovered.

Ovarian cancer has two critical points for therapy. At the

first point, you reduce the tumor though surgery. Essentially, a surgeon removes as much of the tumor as possible without endangering the organs to which the cells adhere. The second point is chemotherapy. The chemotherapy standard is a combination of paclitaxel and carboplatin, the two drugs of choice (as of this writing, anyway). These drugs are given every three weeks for six cycles. At the end of the four to five months, 80 percent of women are in remission. They are tired and live with the looming fear that the cancer might return, but most of them are happy to be alive. Surveillance visits with the doctor occur at three-month intervals for the first year, with the patient undergoing a CA125 test and a pelvic exam each time.

If and when the cancer returns, prognosis is not good. For the average woman with Stage III ovarian cancer, the survival rate at five years is about 30 percent. In other words, if ten women were diagnosed with ovarian cancer, only two to three of them would still be alive five years later. Prognosis is also related to the time it takes for a cancer to recur. The sooner it recurs after completing the initial course of chemotherapy, the poorer the prognosis.

When a woman is diagnosed with a recurrence of ovarian cancer, chemotherapy is restarted. This administration of toxins is now going to be a lifelong process. Each step of the way the woman and her physician together discuss the quality of her life, her willingness to continue chemotherapy and to combat the side effects with which it is associated, and her chances of prolonged survival. Every visit to the doctor is fraught with uncertainty and, yes, terror. *What happens if*

it doesn't work? What's the next step—and is there a next step?
These are the questions the ovarian cancer patient will ask for
the rest of her life—*Is this going to kill me?*—unless she happens to be one of the lucky few whose disease does not recur.
But those lucky few are very few and very far between.

No one really knows why some women with ovarian
cancer live longer than others. Theories include comparisons
of the aggressiveness or thoroughness of the first surgery, basic
intrinsic tumor responsiveness to chemotherapy, sheer luck,
and even, in some very unusual cases, a fortuitous combination of nonprescription supplements. It is true that I have seen
results I can't explain—patients who live beyond all expectations. And I can say with some certainty, albeit unscientific
certainty, that the patients who can still laugh out loud seem
to fare better than those who lose their joie de vivre. Deb was
among those who continued to laugh, but this zest for living
clearly predated the cancer. Perhaps this was true in other
cases. After all, a dour, unhappy woman doesn't suddenly
learn to laugh, and certainly not after being diagnosed with
cancer.

Once a patient's disease recurs, a second-line agent—really
a second *choice* agent—is selected from a multitude of drugs.
Unfortunately, most of these drugs have about a 25 percent
response rate. Each drug works differently, and finding
which drug will work for which woman is a mystery. The
usual course of action is to try a drug, chosen somewhat ran-
domly, for three to four cycles, and then to reevaluate with an
imaging study such as a CT scan. If the agent is working or

even just holding the tumor at bay, which is often the best we can hope for, then we stay with it. If it isn't working, another second-line agent is chosen. This cycle of trial-and-error continues until the therapy's impact on quality of life is adverse enough to consider transitioning to comfort care only.

Sometimes, in the process, people get very, very tired. Chemotherapy is not only an attack on the cancer but also an attack on the body. Fatigue is a major problem for cancer patients. The cause of the fatigue can be anemia, but mostly it is from the constant barrage of toxins. Often the only opportunity for a break is to make a choice to hold off on chemotherapy, but of course this can open the opportunity for the cancer to start growing again in the interim. Another option is hormonal therapy, but most high-grade tumors—which are the tumors most often found in ovarian cancers—tend not to respond to hormonal therapy. Still, if a patient is already exhausted by chemotherapy and chooses not to continue, I've been known to put her on hormones. This type of therapy comes in the form of pills, and it is relatively easy to tolerate. This was what had been done for Deb when she insisted on interrupting her chemotherapy so that she could go Turkey, and it had worked. Then again, maybe it hadn't.

The results of Deb's biopsy came in within twenty-four hours, and our worst fears were confirmed: The cancer had returned. I knew the results before Deb did, but it wasn't my job to share the findings with her. That was up to her principal physicians, Dr. Bouquet or Dr. Darling. By the time I saw her the following day, they'd already broken the news.

"How long do you think I have?" she asked me.

"I really don't know," I told her.

"That's what they said," she remarked vaguely.

She began to talk about her friend Fran Lantz, who had died of ovarian cancer, and who had used total parenteral nutrition to stay alive for the sake of her teenaged child. Deb did not want to go that route. For her, life was very much about quality. With total parenteral nutrition, a patient forgoes food and receives all nutrition by infusion into a vein.

"I'm going to have a stash of drugs squirreled away in the house," she said, repeating what she'd told me earlier. "There's going to come a point where the quality of my life will become unbearable, and at that stage it won't make sense to go on living."

I didn't want to believe it would come to that. She was my friend, and I wasn't yet resigned to her death. As far as I was concerned, the stash was Deb's security blanket. One of the greatest fears for cancer patients is that they will be in tremendous pain, and that their pain will be ignored.

"You're worried about pain?"

"Yes," she said. "Very worried."

"None of us will let you be in pain," I said.

"Promise?"

"Promise."

There were other kinds of pain, of course. Anxiety, fear, and spiritual distress, for example, can produce tremendous physical pain. That's why I talk to my patients, and even try to enlist the help of their friends and families to get them to open up about their fears. Sometimes I get help from chaplains and rabbis, too, but Deb didn't need any of this. She had her family, she had her doctors, and she had me.

As I noted earlier, Deb was being cared for by two medical oncologists, one surgical gynecologic oncologist, one bone marrow specialist, and me. I would be lying if I didn't admit that sometimes I was confused about my role. I was her friend, her doctor, her adviser, and more recently, given the book, her *co-author*. But friend remained at the top of the list.

"I'm not going to prescribe any narcotics," I said. "I'm not going to help you build your 'stash,' as you call it. But when the time comes, I promise I will not let you suffer."

"Is that my friend talking, or my doctor?" she asked.

"It's a good question," I said. "I've been wondering about that myself."

Deb and I had found each other through cancer, and had become intensely close over the years, and now that we were grappling with her mortality, our friendship was turning into an essentially spiritual relationship. I had other patients who had survived well beyond expectations, and it occurred to me that I'd developed increasingly close bonds with them, too. We had the luxury of time—time to talk and to trust and to grow ever closer—but our time was limited, and we knew it. These relationships were intense by definition. If a woman is dying at forty, she has to cram the rest of her natural life—the life that was taken from her—into the little time that's left. Think about that for a moment. It doesn't get much more intense.

I began to notice that some of my fellow oncologists were also being drawn—sometimes against their will—into similarly deep and spiritual relationships. Our patients were living longer and we had time to get to know them as people, not simply as patients. What's more, there was a noticeable power shift in many of these relationships. Where once they had been largely paternalistic, with the doctors making most of the decisions, many of these patients—especially the well-informed ones—were participating actively and aggressively in all of the decisions related to their treatment.

"You know, Lois," Deb told me, "if things go well in the course of one's cancer treatment, one has a long and intense relationship with one's oncologist. If they don't, one has a short and intense relationship with one's oncologist."

She was absolutely right. I looked at her, lying there, knowing she was dying, but I wouldn't allow myself to cry. There would be plenty of time for that later. I was going to move forward—I would be downright *clinical* about this.

"You know, we still have that paper to do," I said.

"Right. Spirituality and ovarian cancer. I haven't forgotten."

"And we have to get back to the book," I said.

"I think I know how it ends," she said, and she smiled.

Several weeks later, Deb developed bowel trouble, followed by a partial obstruction of her kidneys—possibly from a pelvic mass that might have been growing, undetected, while she was in Turkey. Suddenly, we were forced to ask ourselves whether she could live with one kidney, or whether she would need nephrostomy tubes. These are tubes put through the skin of the flank directly into the kidney, and are a way of bypassing the plumbing between the kidney and the bladder. They are then attached to a bag that collects urine. The bag can be worn attached to the leg, possibly under clothes, or simply carried by hand.

I hated the thought of nephrostomy tubes for Deb. She was active. She loved yoga, dancing, movement, *freedom*. The tubes wouldn't be all that limiting, but they would affect how Deb felt about herself, and this could be crippling. It was time to make a quality-of-life decision. Deb had to choose between living with a tube exiting from her back or doing what she needed to do to feel good about herself and her body.

"I can't do it," she said. "I am not going to live with a tube sticking out of my body."

"I understand."

"I'm not going to be medicalized," she said. "I want at least *some* control over my body."

That conversation was a real eye-opener for me. With most patients, I had never really thought of this as a choice: Without the tubes the kidneys wouldn't function. What was there to think about? But when I looked at it from Deb's point of view, I realized that the psychological implications were more far-reaching than I'd imagined. The tubes represented a giant step in the wrong direction—the beginning of a journey into complete *medicalization*.

Fortunately, we consulted a urologist who believed he could fix the problem with stents (internal tubes). Unfortunately, he was only able to place one stent, and we decided that Deb would simply have to make do with one working kidney. I wasn't happy about this, but she really had no other choice.

In the spring, not long after Deb went home, she became disoriented and confused. This was a clear sign of uremia. The single stent had become obstructed, and the kidney was unable to remove the toxins from her system. She was admitted to a hospital in Santa Barbara, where a local urologist not only fixed the problem, but was able to put a stent into the other kidney.

I called Deb after the surgery to see how she felt.

"Well," she said. "I know who I am again."

"That's good," I said.

"And I'm still breathing."

Yes, I thought. *And I'm glad you are.*

8

THE INTERVIEW

On February 24, I got the following e-mail from Deb:

Subject: Abby's sociology of death analysis
        & interview

Lois dear. . . . it's Deb again. I am sending along a paper
and interview Abby did with me for her "sociology
of death" class. . . . I thought it was very thoughtful,
drawing on various theories on the process of dying
that she has encountered this quarter. I cannot imagine that you will have time to read it now, but perhaps
some time later.

    You need to email me so that I know you and yours
are ok and that you are not put out with my inability to
do social science research. Love Deb

. . .

Abby was kind enough to share the interview and the paper with me, and parts of it, slightly abbreviated. After asking the standard interview-opening question about age and ethnicity—which Deb, in true form, laughed her way through ("I be a Jewish white girl!")—Abby dove straight into the heart of the matter.

Abby's analysis of their interview was so wonderfully moving and insightful. Her introspection and maturity clearly comforting as well as inspiring to Deb. It was then, I thought, that Abby really would be "O.K." Of her mother, Abby wrote,

Death is an aggressor. Deb alludes to this when she describes facing cancer and thereby death as wanting to "face the fucker" and "beat the shit out of it." She is attacking death because she sees death as attacking her. Deb felt this way most intensely when she was first diagnosed, but with the passage of time has come an ability to manage her anger, grief, and anxiety from day to day.

To live in a state of perpetual anxiety is to not truly live at all. Much of life was like that for Deb, until she underwent a bone marrow transplant. Her experience of "dying and rising again" instilled in her a sense that what enlivened her was the same substance that enlivened the world. She then felt that her illness, and what would be her subsequent death, was not a personal attack, but rather a continuation of the course of all life. This does not mean that Deb is now comfortable with dying; rather she vacillates between several different coping strategies to maintain emotional stability in her day-to-day life. [Stephen] Levine expounds culti-

vating "an openness to death," but for Deb it was too difficult to remain open to the unknown, to the thought of leaving, and when she maintained that mind-set, she often became terribly depressed (Kastenbaum, 25). She could not balance her chemotherapy, job, relationships, and emotional self unless she maintained a bit of distance on death. Deb compartmentalizes in order to remain a participant in the world around her; she "responds to some aspects of [death]" but does not connect, or think about the details, the actuality of when she will die (Kastenbaum, 38). In this way, she can talk about death with her family and face death alone, but she is able to maintain control over when she accesses those emotions."

I don't know that there's much I can add to the interview. Abby's ability to look at her mother, to put aside both her own fear and pain, and look into the deeper roots of Deb's attitude toward her own life and impending death was more than impressive. She put into words—beautiful, concrete words—underlying themes and issues that, in her place, I might have been hard put to face.

My own life was moving in a completely different direction. By this point, Nuri and I had put both our houses on the market, found a wonderful new home on a man-made lake, and decided to get married the following April.

One of the big issues—outside of the guest list, the caterers, the flowers, the seating arrangements, the location, and just about everything else—was the question of *who* was going to marry us. We were from wildly different cultures, but at heart we were one, so we decided to use the services of a Unitarian Universalist minister, a woman we were both very fond of. I also asked Deb if she would say a few words at our ceremony, and she said she'd be honored.

In December 2004, Deb made the promised trip to Houston for our joint lecture. In the preceding weeks, as we'd prepared for it, we had agreed to use a standard PowerPoint lecture outline, based on our joint paper, which I later hoped to publish in one of the medical journals.

When I saw Deb and Giles in the lobby of the convention location that day, she was as elegantly dressed as ever, but it was immediately clear that much had changed. She was skinny, pale, and tired, and she immediately informed me that she'd been unable to tolerate anything but liquids—mostly hot tea.

"Well, to be completely honest, you don't look too good," I said. "Are you sure you're up for this?"

"I'm fine," she said. "Don't worry about a thing."

She threw up shortly before the talk, but moments later we found ourselves standing in front of several hundred oncologists and oncology nurses, some of whom had come from overseas to hear us talk. We plunged in, taking turns, and the presentation took the form of a dialogue.

"It should not be surprising to any of you that cancer survivors as a group are generally a grateful crowd," I began. "The form that gratitude takes is varied—everything from gifts and food, to book dedications, to financial contributions to those institutions that do cancer work. Patient gratitude also often takes religious forms: prayers, testimonials, spiritual autobiographies, and narratives that invoke the divine and the human encounter with the absolute. In a nation that self-consciously finds itself under God's protection, it should not be surprising that those who have at least imaginatively encountered their own mortality would express their sense of wonder, in religious and spiritual terms, to the healers who work so diligently to save lives."

As we talked, we showed slides of a number of Mark Rothko paintings, many of which are extremely spiritual in nature. We discussed the scientific and medical community's renewed interest in spirituality—the Mind Body Institute at Harvard Medical School was cited as an example—and we tried to provide a definition of spirituality that might work for everyone.

When Deb stepped up to the microphone, the energy in the audience visibly sharpened. "Cancer," she said slowly, "causes a confrontation of limits. For some it is a state of shock. You experience this as—a *recognizing* that there is something in you that has the capability of destroying you." She paused to let that sink in. Her hands, gripping the podium, were thin and frail, but her voice was strong and quiet.

"Earlier on in my diagnosis," she told us, "I experienced cancer as a kind of 'other'—and it was better that way because I thought I could beat it, that I could *beat* this fucker. Knowing what I know now—that it will eventually overtake me—it is a different way of living with it than when I was living in that in-between life, when I thought maybe we could kill it and I would be done with it." She cleared her throat. "It is part of me now; it is my dharma, the life I am living. It is the life I have—it is my way of going."

It was an honest, almost naked account of her reconciliation to her cancer and her death. The audience was silent as I stepped back to the microphone to continue the discussion.

We talked about aging Baby Boomers, and how they seemed to be getting more religious with the passage of time. And we even talked about Sir James Frazer, author of *The Golden Bough*, who nearly a hundred years ago argued that religion was simply a *stage* in human development—a point on which, clearly, he'd been very wrong.

Finally, we closed with an interesting statistic: Between 1980 and 1982, only about one hundred scientific articles were published on religion and medicine. Between 2000 and 2002, the number climbed to eleven hundred.

When we were done, Deb was so exhausted that she retired with Giles to her hotel room, assuring me that she was fine. She wasn't fine, but she made it fine.

Writing together and speaking on issues related to human spirituality and cancer care have provided me with the opportunity to enjoy what my mother would have called "the pleasure of her company." It has also enabled me to reflect on the character of human friendship and the ways in which friendship shapes the present and informs the future. Dr. Lois has helped to keep me in the world, not because she has managed the diagnostic tests or the chemotherapy agents that are involved in a bone marrow transplant or in the cancer care that followed when again I fell out of the Remission Society. Rather, I am younger for her friendship, and with her I have plans that involve both desire and good work, the imaginary and the real.

Dr. Lois and I have traveled to Paris together, spoken at international ovarian conferences together, and adventured in Istanbul with my husband and her fiancé. I would not have met her apart from ovarian cancer and, strange to say, my life is better for her friendship. She has opened a world of women and science, medicine, and real work that before entering the cancer community I had no inkling about.

Not long after she returned to Santa Barbara, I received a cryptic e-mail from her:

Lois, I had a dream about you and Nuri the night before last and the two of you were driving around in a blue MG sports car, happy, excited, and with a number of places to see. Is this a honeymoon?

She was also writing frequent e-mails to Abby, a few of which follow:

Abby, you are a very deep person and I don't claim to have any real insight into the state of your own reflective pool. Yikes Abby, I am just being foolish here, so very happy to hear from you . . .

I had a long talk with Lois this morning as she prepares herself and her daughter and Nuri and the rest of us for the nuptials at the end of the month. I will be delivering a blessing of some sort. Any ideas?

I hope to do some dancing at Lois and Nuri's wedding . . .

Hello dearie. . . . So wonderful to hear your voice first thing in the morning and to be reminded that I also heard it last thing last night. Ah, conscience and conscientiousness—it is elusive and channeled through the lace of Ambien and Paxil and all the rest. Having lived such a drug-free life through the early years, it is interesting to come to the world of drugs and to embrace them now. The lesson in all of this is not to be too judgmental about almost everything. I will however draw the line at adultery and murder—I think. More on this later perhaps.

I am trying to get organized here before I leave for Houston, and I find myself thinking more and more about my talk at the coming marriage. I can't reach Lois on the phone and of course I don't want to either bore people or offend the couple. I did get Lois a silk "Frida Kahlo" scarf, though.

Dancing, which I hope to do a good deal of at Lois's wedding, remains one of the great human endeavors.

Nuri and I were married on April 30, 2005, at the Mariposa Ranch, a beautiful little bed-and-breakfast outside Houston, where we took over the main house and several of the outlying cottages. My parents came, of course, as did my grandmother, along with my sister and her entire family. Nuri's brother came from Dubai. Nuri's mother was unable to come due to the difficulty of travel from the occupied territories. And of course Deb and Giles came.

Nuri wore a tan suit and I wore a midlength cream-colored dress with spaghetti straps, and a silk, fringed, embroidered shawl—a gift from Deb. Jessica, in a flowered dress, looked absolutely beautiful.

Before the ceremony got under way, our friend Paul Klemperer, a musician, mingled with the guests, playing jazzy tunes on his saxophone. When he stopped playing, that was my cue, and I walked out with Jessica. Nuri was waiting up ahead, with the minister. It had thundered and rained the night before, and the ground was cool and damp.

My sister and her husband, along with Nuri's brother, sister, and niece, read selected poems, and then it was Deb's turn.

"To begin," she said, "I want to speak about Lois and Nuri's work in the world. It is different in kind, but strangely similar in its trajectory and its goods. Both are involved in the renewal, the restoration, the repair, literally the healing—*Tikkun ha olam*—the healing of the world.

"They recognize both their foreignness to each other and their fundamental kinship. Both are engaged in repairing the world and enlarging it for us." She spoke very eloquently about the differing worlds we'd come from, and how both of us were healers and unifiers, crossing cultural boundaries, in our working lives. It seemed natural, she said, that together we should make a cosmopolitan world to live in.

She continued:

"Lois really does cure cancer and, when she can't, she eases the journey for her patients. Her work at Anderson has brought her healing touch to the poor, to immigrants and, as she will tell you, to the uncooperative.

"A healer in a hurry, Lois's moral vision and her extraordinary élan for living permeate the whole of her life and times and inform the quality of her relationships with the women under her care, their families, and her colleagues. This élan also shapes her feelings for her own family, particularly her primordial love, her mother-love for daughter, Jessie, even as it enlivens the community of friends she has created throughout the world.

"Nuri, born in Jerusalem, raised in Ramallah, educated in Istanbul, a lover of things Scots, is a true cosmopolitan, a citizen of the world. His work, like Lois's, concerns itself with renewal, repair, and restoration.

"In his case, it is the repair of the artistic fabric that weaves human communities together. Most obviously, we see it at Anderson where he actually links the worlds of cancer care together.

"We also see it in his work as an artist and translator of the cultural traditions of art that render American folk music—

the blues—accessible and understandable to a contemporary audience.

"It is an extraordinary act of the imagination. Nuri is able to forge links that cross cultural boundaries and to demonstrate the ways in which American folk music invokes the nearly universal human dramas of suffering, loss, death and desire.

"It is not surprising that, together, Lois and Nuri have created a cosmopolitan world community in the life they have made.

"As their family and friends, we recognize that we are all bigger and better for the requirements their life together makes on us. And of course, it is a site for a great deal of fun. Laughter, conversation, and good food, and music are the structural supports of a life full of love, passion, vision and renewal.

"To fulfill the second part of my charge—to say something about what their marriage might mean to Lois and Nuri—I want to quote two of my favorite sources on how to be married: the Book of Ecclesiastes from the Hebrew Bible and author and mystery story writer Carolyn Heilbrun.

"Heilbrun's advice may appear more opaque and reflects the contemporary experience of a two-career home, with kids and a dog. For her, and for American philosopher and musician Stanley Cavell, all happy marriages are really remarriages. Good marriages are always in the process of re-creating, revising, restoring, if you will, the original marriage.

"There are no public trophies and it's not obvious to the observer who's in charge. It is more like a Balanchine ballet than a petit pas de deux."

Deb closed her speech with a passage from Ecclesiastes,

4–9: "Two are better than one, because they have a good reward for their toil. For if they fall one will lift up his fellow: but woe to him who is alone when he falls and has not another to lift him up. Again, if two lie together, they are warm; but how can one be warm alone? And though a man might prevail against one who is alone, two will withstand him. A threefold cord is not quickly broken."

We had written our own vows. Nuri went first:

"Lois, over three years ago on a sunny Sunday afternoon, I found myself at a festival on stage introducing bands, and I noticed an attractive woman attending to her daughter in a way that reminded me of family and how families should be. I knew then you had qualities I have long waited for."

When it was my turn, I said, in part: "Nuri, you had been in my life long before I laid eyes on you. Sometimes I think it was fate that we met, united by the Gypsies. You are the most generous, most loving, kindest man I have ever met. You have the ability to get excited by life through your senses and to make me laugh and enjoy my life. In so many ways, you have connected me to a world bigger than my own."

After we exchanged rings, Nuri addressed Jessica directly: "Jessica, I love your Mommy and today we are married. I want you to know I love you dearly as well. We have had many special times together, being silly, going to festivals, watching your recitals, traveling the world from Dubai to Austin to New Jersey, and especially watching you grow into the wonderful person you have become. I know we will have many more happy times together, you, your Mommy, and me, and I look forward to becoming a parent you can always trust and confide in. I am honored to officially become part of this wonderful family; I am also thrilled you and your mother are joining the Nuri family."

At that point, the two of us gave Jessica a small gift—a circular gold necklace with silver flecks that sparkled when they caught the light. Jessica then read a poem called "Family Ties," by Timothy Lennox.

When it was over, musician Seth Walker took the stage. His band is from Austin and plays blues with a touch of New Orleans. Everyone was in a dancing mood, including Deb. It was great to see her so happy and so full of life.

It was also great to see my father happy. Much as he liked Nuri, he had been concerned that our cultural differences were insurmountable, but by evening's end it was clear his fears had been allayed. We partied well into the night, and in the wee hours we found ourselves sitting around a bonfire. My mother and Nuri both picked up guitars and sang folk songs. Many others had also brought guitars and began playing along. I looked at the surrounding faces and saw the dancing flames reflected in their faces. Muslims, Jews, Christians, nonbelievers—present together as a community.

I looked over at Nuri. In marrying him, I had gone from a predictable, provincial, and somewhat tentative view of life to a more global perspective of the world and how I fit into it. More important, he was still patiently teaching me to enjoy the present—to make the most of every moment. As Deb would say, I was a lucky girl!

When we returned to normal life, I tried to find time to work on the book, but I was busy and made little progress.

In July, Deb flew to Tokyo to visit Abby, who had been studying at the University of California, Irvine, and was doing a semester abroad. Abby had been reluctant to leave California, fearing for Deb's health, but both Deb and Giles had urged her to go, even promising to try to visit, since Giles had been invited to meet with some old friends from Kyoto. As it turned out, Deb became fairly ill, so Kyoto should have been out of the question, but she decided she would make the trip anyway to spend time with Abby. She later told me that the visit was one of the happiest times of her life. She and Abby ate, talked, explored the city, and one wild night found themselves at a karaoke bar, singing their hearts out. Their repertoire included "I Need a Hero," by Bonnie Tyler, "Don't Leave Me This Way," by Thelma Houston (among others), and Rod Stewart's inimitable "Maggie May."

In September, I wrote Deb to tell her that Nuri and I were thinking of going to Ramallah to visit his mother. I also told her about our recent move into our new home, and that we'd done some volunteer work on behalf of victims of Hurricane Katrina.

Hi Deb!

How are you feeling?

The book is going slow—are you still writing?

We are spending every waking moment unpacking or

doing 4th grade homework (anything outside of working on the book, that is).

The house is SO BEAUTIFUL! I love it! I can't
wait for you to come—the guest room is done!

I have worked on our draft—I removed some,
added some, and tried to organize it better. See what
you think.

I need to visit you but am still considering Ramallah in October.

I will send you my part of the book to date soon.

Houston is interesting—I volunteered at the Convention Center, not at the Astrodome yet. Nuri volunteered at the Astrodome—helped do computer
searches and find people—for 8 hours!

I on the other hand am so subspecialized that I was
essentially useless as a physician!

Love and miss you,

Lois

Two months later, in October 2005, Nuri and I left for
Ramallah. He hadn't been there since the summer his father
died, and he wanted to see his mother to make sure she was
managing on her own. The trip got off to a very rocky start,
to say the least.

Well Deb—This has been quite an experience. I am
writing from Tel Aviv—Nuri is still with his mom.
However, he is in Amman.

They detained him, 10 hours in Tel Aviv. Regardless of his American passport, to the Israelis he will always be a Palestinian, and now can never travel through Tel Aviv. They essentially put him in jail and made me enter the transit lounge. We were separated from 9am, when our flight arrived, until 7pm, when we were able to catch a Royal Jordanian plane to Jordan (only one or two phone calls were allowed). It was terrible for both of us, but especially for Nuri, and a huge disappointment. We flew to Jordan with plans to cross on the King Hussein Bridge, but because he did not have an updated Jordanian passport or a Palestinian passport (which he has never had) he could not enter [Israel]. We spent all our time in Amman. We spent three of the days getting there or planning our departure. Nuri still doesn't have a flight out—he has to buy a whole new ticket from Amman. He will never be able to go to Jerusalem despite it being his birth place (his entire family's birth place) and the home of his mother and aunt for the majority of their lives. As for me, I have been treated much better on the return flight, without him. I was still searched completely but much less rudely than on the way in. I never made it to Israel unless you count the overnight last night after my flight back on Royal Jordanian.

All was not lost, however. Nuri's mom worried about us a lot by day three and crossed with a Palestinian permit to Amman. I met his mother, his aunt, uncle, cousins and they were all wonderful! His uncle owns a small hotel in Amman and reminded me of my own grandfather—a funny, intellectual old man! Second bad luck was that Ramadan happened on the second day—all restaurants closed during the day (eating only in hotels, instead of his mother's home-cooked meals). His uncle's hotel makes a good lamb dish and I ate that three times!

On day four we convinced his mother (in her 70s) to go with us to the Dead Sea. We went overnight to a resort and had a lovely time. I heard all about her life and of course she likes me—really does, I think. I like her very much, too. We floated and got covered in mud. Beautiful trip. We also went to Mount Nebo but as for sight-seeing that was it, unless of course you count seeing Israel from the other side of the Dead Sea. What a trip!

I miss Nuri already and I know I really do love him! Israel feels funny as kind of an outsider. Lots to talk about. More later. Hope you and Giles are well—perhaps Ramallah next year.

Love, Lois

The experience was far worse than I'd described it. When we were at the airport in Tel Aviv, I protested to the Israeli authorities, "But Nuri is my husband, and he has been a U.S. citizen for twenty years. He is the nicest man in the world and he just wants to visit his mom!"

It didn't help. He was taken to a jail cell to wait for the next flight out, and I waited for the same flight in the airport. When they announced the flight, almost ten hours later, Nuri was nowhere in sight. I was one of the last to board, and he still wasn't there. I was a nervous wreck. I sat in the plane, trying not to hyperventilate, and the flight attendants did their best to comfort me. Finally, just before takeoff, they brought Nuri onto the plane. I threw my arms around him, and all the passengers gave us a hearty round of applause.

The trip ended well, however. Since we couldn't go into Ramallah, as I noted in my letter to Deb, Nuri's mother came to see us in Amman. She was seventy-six years old and had to walk across the bridge by herself.

One day, we took her with us to a hotel on the Dead Sea. We sat outside, on a huge, tented balcony, talking well into the evening. We could see all the way across the water, to Jericho. She told me about growing up in Jerusalem with three sisters and two brothers, and about the beloved dog she had as a child. She talked about the war of 1967, describing the bombed and burned-out buildings and the white surrender flags in the windows, many of them charred by the flames. Nuri remembered the flags.

The next day, we went into the market and she bought me a beautiful necklace. The quoted price was very high, but she was a great negotiator and refused to budge until they accepted her offer.

I also met Nuri's uncle, a charming, sophisticated man. He sat down and had a glass of wine with me. "If you read the Koran, it doesn't say you shouldn't drink," he told me. "It says you shouldn't pray if you're drunk." After he finished his wine, he looked over at Nuri, who had a fuzzy little soul-patch at the time. "Let me ask you," he said. "You are a doctor. Is there any way to remove that ugly thing from under my nephew's lip?"

Soon after we returned to the States, I discovered I was pregnant, and I immediately called Deb to share the good news. She was overjoyed, but a little sad, too. "I'm not going to be around to meet her," she said.

Suddenly, I began to think about all the things I was going to miss about Deb. Her smile. Those crazy, ever-changing eyeglasses. The wild, multicolored socks she was partial to. Her red, patent-leather Dansko clogs. I would miss the jewelry she wore—the rings and the clanking bracelets—and I would miss her contagious laugh. I would miss the way she liked to sit in her big chair, with her fuzzy socks and her cup of hot tea, a book resting on her lap. And I would miss the way she always greeted me, with that big smile and so much energy: "Good morning, Lois!"

Now, having spoken to her, I realized that she was right—she wouldn't be around to enrich the life of my second child, as she'd done with Jessie.

I missed her already.

9

THE GREAT UNKNOWN

In January, Deb returned to Houston for more tests. Unfortunately, the news was grim. The latest chemotherapy combination was not working. The CT scans showed some spots on her liver and lungs that had not been there previously, and her CA125 level had more than doubled since her last visit.

The day after the tests, all of our worst fears were confirmed, and Deb was as crushed as I'd ever seen her. Giles himself was in tears, and really—what was there to say?

They were scheduled to leave for California the next day, but I asked Deb to stay with me at my place.

"I need to be home with my things," she said.

"Your things will wait," I replied. I hated the thought of her alone at the beach house while Giles was at work. I thought a few days to process the bad news, with a friend at her side, would do her a world of good. "I'm giving another lecture on spirituality, and I could really use your help."

She wasn't listening because she was crushed. This diagnosis was too much for her, and she was thinking about what lay ahead.

"Am I going to be in a lot of pain?" she asked.

"It's different for everyone," I said.

"Tell me what I can expect."

I told her. Usually, with ovarian cancer, the bowels stop working, so the patient will eat but the food won't move through her system. She'll start to feel bloated, and nauseated, and eventually she would grow weak from lack of nourishment. At that stage, most patients tend to sleep a lot.

"What about pain?" she asked again.

"We'll give you morphine. And you'll get a pump, so you can use it as needed."

"Am I going to live to see Abby graduate from college?"

"I don't know, Deb. I wish I could answer that, but I honestly don't know. June is a long way off."

"I don't know what to say," she said, looking as forlorn as I'd ever seen her.

"Deb, I don't want you going home like this. I'm giving a talk in a few days, January 12, my birthday. And I want you to do this with me." The talk was on spirituality and caregiving, and I had prepared it at the urging of the Advanced Practice nurses at M. D. Anderson. "I could really use your help with it," I said. I meant it, too. I also knew it would help take her mind off the bad news.

"What do you think happens to us when we die, Lois?"

"I don't know," I said. "I thought that was your department."

"Do you think we come back in one form or another, or is that wishful thinking?"

"I'd like to think we come back."

"Maybe we only live on in the memories of others."

"Maybe," I said. "And maybe that's not so bad."

The next day, Deb's doctors started her on Vidaisa, a newly approved chemotherapy agent that had shown promise with solid tumors. She left the hospital and moved in with Nuri and Jessica and me, and Giles came with her. He could only stay two nights, but Deb promised to stay for the presentation.

In the beginning, I hadn't really known Giles all that well. He had, I felt, always seen me as a doctor—as part of the Anderson experience—while Deb saw me primarily as a friend. But after so many trips to California and their visits when Deb was in Houston for her regular evaluations, Giles and I had gotten to know each other pretty well; on this trip we grew a little closer. He was a serious and sensitive man whose approach to life had always seemed a little academic, but now his emotions were taking over. He was deeply worried about losing Deb, and I sensed that he also in some ways feared what his life would be like without her.

One evening, when Deb was asleep, Giles and I went for a walk around the lake. "How much time does she have?" he asked.

"Deb asked me the same question, and I honestly don't know."

Giles had been the caregiver from the very start, and his job wasn't over yet. Worse lay ahead, and he knew it. It is the same with people who care for Alzheimer's patients. The illness takes over your life, and there are times when the anxiety and the waiting are almost more than one can bear. I remembered Shirley, the girl Deb had told me about, who greeted the news of her mother's passing with a "strange smile."

"But you must have an estimate?" Giles asked.

"It's hard to tell. As long as she can poop, breathe, and eat, it's impossible to predict."

"And if she stops eating?"

"Weeks, probably."

"What about feeding her though an IV?"

"If there's a specific, reachable goal—a wedding, a graduation—then you might want to consider it. But it's more complicated than it seems. There are a lot of risks connected to intravenous nutrition, and I'm not sure she'll consider it. She's still very conscious of how Fran looked at the end."

"I feel like Ishmael feels in the opening pages of *Moby-Dick*," Giles said. "'Grim about the mouth.'"

After he left for the airport, I sat with Deb for a while. "I am sure Giles is going to remarry," she said. "He's a great catch. Some young woman in his department will find him.

He has never been alone. He went from his mom to his first wife, and from his first wife to me. He will make someone very happy after I'm gone. He made me very happy."

It was all I could do not to cry.

After I left Deb's room, I dug up my old copy of *Moby-Dick* to see precisely what Giles had been referring to. The passage he had cited was on the very first page: "Whenever I find myself growing grim about the mouth; whenever it is a damp, drizzly November in my soul; whenever I find myself involuntarily pausing before coffin warehouses, and bringing up the rear of every funeral I meet; and especially whenever my hypos get such an upper hand of me, that it requires a strong moral principle to prevent me from deliberately stepping into the street and methodically knocking people's hats off—then, I account it high time to get to sea as soon as I can." Giles clearly wasn't interested in lighting out, but I could see how the passage reflected his own anger and sense of desolation.

For the next few days, when I wasn't in the hospital, Deb and I focused on our joint presentation. But we also worked on the book. I remember the two of us sitting on the couch in my living room, each of us typing away on our laptops, pausing now and then to read aloud to each other. At one point, Deb said, "We're going to have to talk about the ending. I don't want it to be depressing—I don't want it to end with my death."

"Okay," I said.

"I'd like it to end with the birth of your daughter."

Nuri and I had already picked out our daughter's name: Leila Rose. Rose was Deb's middle name.

On my way to the hospital later that same day, I called my sister Karen and told her about my conversation with Deb. I cried but managed to pull myself together. This wasn't what Deb needed from me. I told myself I could get through it. I talked to patients about death every day, sometimes three or four times a day, and I generally managed to end the talks on a note that provided some degree of hope—some reachable goal. I would do the same for Deb, I told myself. We had too much to do to allow ourselves to be sad.

When I got back to the house, she told me she'd been on the phone with her son, Adam, who was getting married in December. "I won't be around for the wedding," she said. "I won't be around for Abby's graduation. I won't be part of your life or Jessica's life and I'm not even going to meet Leila Rose."

I said nothing.

"I'm wearing out, Lois," she continued. "I'm not going to be around much longer, and it makes me sad. I really don't want to leave this place."

It was the first time we had acknowledged her death with that level of directness, and we found ourselves talking, once again, about the Great "Distinguished Thing." My Catholic grandmother often talked of heaven, convinced that our extended family was all up there, in human form, smiling down at us. "She was convinced they would be there to greet her when the time came," I said.

"What about your mother?"

"She hedges her bets," I said. "She'll say, 'Nobody knows what happens, but I hope it's wonderful.'"

Even Deb, a professor of comparative religion, didn't have any solid answers, but she felt, just as I did, that life couldn't simply *end*. Our élan vital had to go somewhere, right? It didn't seem possible that that energy, that life force—our *souls,* if you will—would simply be extinguished. And while neither of us believed in reincarnation, we both felt that death is a transition to some sort of larger whole.

I believed that then, and I believe it to this day. I think that when we die our energy rejoins the world as a freer, formless, global spirit, sustaining the continuum. I believed this even as a child, and because I believed it I decided never to be buried. How could I rejoin the world if I was put away in a box and buried in a hole in the ground? No, that wasn't for me. I would be cremated, and my ashes would become part of the visible, living earth.

As Deb and I talked about this, Jessica came into the room, and Deb reached for the King James Bible she'd been leafing though earlier that day. It occurred to me that she and I had never talked directly about God.

Deb proceeded to read from Isaiah, the same section she said she'd read many years earlier, at the funeral of a close friend who had committed suicide: "'The voice said, Cry. And he said, What shall I cry? All flesh is grass, and all the goodliness thereof is as the flower of the field.'"

"All flesh is grass," I repeated.

"Yes," she said. "Isn't that exactly what we've been talking about?"

On the day of our joint presentation, Deb and I met outside the lecture hall. She looked very elegant, as always, sitting there drinking her hot tea, but she was solemn.

Nuri had arranged to have the lecture taped, and the three of us went into the hall and watched him set up the video equipment. The room filled up with nurses, and the presentation got under way.

Deb and I opened with a reference to Sigmund Freud's definition of spirituality: "An oceanic sense of boundlessness and oneness between the ego and the outside world." We spoke about transcendence—the feeling that we were all connected to something larger than ourselves—and about the way religious rituals help imbue our lives with meaning, whether in childbirth, marriage, or death.

In the context of the hospital, we noted, spirituality is about relationships in the face of life-threatening illness. It is about touch, listening, and accepting uncertainty, and it is about our desire to uncover deeper truths beneath the surface. "Spirituality is also about doing everything we can for our fellow human beings, even as we recognize that there are things we cannot change," I said.

When Deb spoke about her relationships with her nurses and her doctors, and how much they had meant to her, the room became very still. Everyone was aware that they were in the presence of a woman who wasn't long for the world.

After the presentation, Deb and Nuri and I went out to an Italian restaurant for dinner, and everything felt tinged with sadness. The next morning, without saying much, Deb flew home.

The moment she left, I realized I still hadn't come to terms with the fact that I was really losing her. We had talked about it, yes, but I was in denial. I didn't want to believe that she was really leaving. There would be no more conversations. No more shopping expeditions. No trips abroad. No more listening to her big laugh or basking in her palpable glow. And I'd never, ever get to sit in on one of her classes.

Deb called from Santa Barbara the next day. "I called the school," she said. "I told them I wouldn't be back in the fall."

"I'm so sorry," I said.

"My chairman was very nice, but it was hard on him. He said it made him very sad, and he sounded it. He's going to take my big class. And my other two classes—well, I'll do them for a little while, but that's not going to last."

"Are you okay?" I asked. It was a feeble question, and she ignored it.

"I want to die by myself," she said. "Lying in my hammock in my backyard, listening to the sound of the waves and playing Mozart—*loudly,* to disturb the neighbors."

"Okay," I said.

"Giles has other ideas," she went on. "He wants to be by my side with Adam and Abby. But that doesn't appeal to me.

I don't want to become weaker and weaker. I don't want to see myself that way, and I don't want others to see me that way. I'll just lie there in the hammock, alone, feeling the sun on my tired bones, and I'll take my drugs and go to sleep."

"If that's what you want, you have my full support," I said.

"They are participating, but it's really me, you know. You die alone."

"I know," I said, but I'm not sure she heard me.

"I watched Fran die," she reminded me. "She looked so small and weak. I really don't want to look like that."

I didn't say anything. I didn't know what to say.

"Do you think I'll be able to take my stash?" she asked. "I say I will, but who knows what I'll do when the time comes?"

"I want to fly to Santa Barbara in April to work on our book," I said. "How does that sound?"

"It sounds lovely," she said. Then she was quiet.

10

THE DISTINGUISHED THING

When I was diagnosed for a second time, I couldn't even register it, not even the name. I just felt, Well, that's it. And when they had this treatment to offer, I was very surprised. The second diagnosis sort of took the wind out of me.

I think when they told us about the second cancer, Giles and I both knew the end was soon. It wasn't anything they said. They had ideas of what we could do. But we just felt it was done. There was a reality to it that we had been able to avoid before. So then it was that the Vidaisa shots in the stomach immediately started.

Why did we go ahead and try it? It had everything to do with Dr. Bouquet. He really wanted me to try it, but I never understood *why. I wondered why he didn't just want to stop. He told us it could help, could work, and could give me more time for the graduation and the wedding. So that was the thinking. By the third night, I started vomiting. It came on me in a splash. There was no lead up to the vomit—it was just vomit.*

At that point, I had to talk to my colleagues and tell them I couldn't teach, and to make new arrangements for others to teach my classes. My chairman took over my big class, I took two others, but I am done with them now, I think. The big deal for me was having to tell the college that I wouldn't be back in the fall. I had to tell the dean. He was very sweet. He just said it was all "so sad." He was very lovely. It was all he needed to say. He said he would take care of it and that was it.

But then my body took over, strange things started happening, my face got infected, and I didn't feel very well. That is the interesting question, When is enough enough? *For my dear Fran, it was never enough. It was her doctor who said, "Fran, I've got nothing left to give you." Of course, her desire to continue was due to her son.*

So what now?

We had intended to end this book with the birth of Leila Rose, Lois's daughter. We didn't want the book to be a stereotypical drama ending with the death of the Beloved Patient, but there are some things over which you have very little control. So come to find out, it is a story about the death of the Beloved Patient.

When a cancer drama begins, one is overwhelmed by the fear of dying, and the trade-off with treatment is really a pact with the devil. The patient is willing to "enjoy" a kind of living, not the living to which he or she is accustomed. Gradually, over the course of my almost nine-year encounter with ovarian cancer, the formula for living has changed. Death is something to be feared, but it is also a source of comfort, rest, and release. Many years ago, after a dear friend tried to fly home from the top of a Seattle bridge, I read from Isaiah at her funeral. It is perhaps the most expressive sense of being welcomed home after a very difficult journey. Honestly, death is very often the solution of the human drama and offers a patient and her family the prospect of ease, comfort, and peace.

In late March, I sent Deb a draft of the book, incorporating everything she had sent me, and hoped she would feel strong enough to work on it. I wasn't optimistic, however. Since her return to Santa Barbara, Deb had been admitted to the hospital three times. The first time, not surprisingly, was after the first cycle of the new chemotherapy. I can always tell by the lack of communication, unanswered e-mails, absence of phone calls, and unanswered cell phone that something has happened. She developed an infection and was admitted for intravenous antibiotics. This infection wiped her out beyond anything that was expected. This event, taken in light of months of anemia and low white blood cell counts unresponsive to therapy, led Dr. Sun to diagnose Deb with a rare form of leukemia called myelodysplastic syndrome (MDS). Deb and Giles flew back to Houston for a two- to three-day visit for a bone marrow biopsy, and, alas, the diagnosis was confirmed.

The visit to Houston was strangely short, and I barely got a chance to see her. But I understood. They were grieving together; it was not my time to grieve. Giles was very protective of Deb. He arranged appointments, spoke to her various doctors, accompanied her on all her visits, and kept visitors at bay. I wished I could have been there for her, but this wasn't about me.

They left abruptly, with time only for a quick goodbye. I felt isolated, but there really wasn't anything I could have said or done that would have helped. I know very little about leukemia or the treatments associated with it. Oncologists often separate themselves into what are called oncologists of "liquid" tumors, such as leukemia and lymphoma, and "solid" tumors, the ones measurable by substance and by size.

From this point on, things got steadily worse. Deb was again hospitalized, a very short time later, for renal complications. Her creatinine, a measure of her kidney function, was rising, and she was unable to stay hydrated. She also had an upper respiratory tract infection—not her first—and sounded terrible on the phone, but she seemed to be recovering. Two days later I talked with Giles. He said Deb had become disoriented and had a fever, and that she'd been readmitted to the hospital.

When she got home, she called me. "This isn't what I expected," she told me. She was demoralized and exhausted. "How long can this go on?"

I let her rest, but she called me again later that evening. "You know, Lois," she said, sounding more lucid than she had earlier. "I've had enough . . . I wanted to watch Abby graduate, and I wanted to be there for Adam's wedding, but I'm not going to make it. But you know something? They're both going to be just fine. I could have died five years ago. Abby still needs me, but not in the same way she needed me back then, when she was so angry at me for being sick. I look at her now and I know she's going to be okay. *Better* than okay. She really is a terrific human being."

Deb drifted a little, becoming disoriented and incoherent at times. She was short of breath and clearly very tired. "I am so happy for Adam, and so proud of him," she said finally. "DeAnn is a wonderful girl. I can see how happy she makes him. I'm glad he found someone who's crazy about him."

The next week I was in Palm Springs, California, for a gynecologic oncology conference. I called the second day of the conference to see how Deb was doing. She was in the hospital, and she sounded very weak. "I'm thinking of coming out to see you in two or three weeks," I told her. I was six months pregnant and I didn't think I'd be in any shape to travel beyond then.

"I might not be around in two or three weeks," Deb said.

I called Giles for details and he said that she had taken a very bad turn.

"I don't want to interfere," I said. "I know this is about the family, not about me."

"No," he said. "If you can get away, it would mean a lot to us."

I called Nuri. I was missing him and Jessica, but I told him I needed to see Deb.

I made the four-hour drive north to Santa Barbara, listening to a Beatles marathon on the radio and crying. I kept thinking of how lucky I was to know Deb, and how the people who didn't know her would be the poorer for it. She was such a giving person. So full of life. So interested in her fellow human beings. I had never met anyone with such a knack for *seeing* others. Whether it was a nurse, or a hospital grounds-keeper, or a waiter in a restaurant—Deb was intensely curious about who they were and what made them tick. Most of us are lost in that bottomless black hole of self-absorption, but not Deb—Deb's curiosity about her fellow human beings was insatiable. What's more, she had a habit of trying to find the best in everyone, and when she found it she dug deep. Deb was always looking for the qualities that defined people, that made each of us different, and she was intensely curious about how those qualities had developed in that particular person, and how they had affected the way they saw the world. She was interested in the forces that shaped each human life, the qualities that made each of us unique.

This was a form of religion, I guess. *Who are we? How do we become the people we become? What does it all add up to? And what happens to us when we're gone?*

I stood next to the bed and reached for her hand. She barely had the strength to squeeze it. In a voice that was barely a notch above a whisper, she said, "I didn't even get to sixty."

She was fifty-six years old. It seemed horribly unfair.

"The only reason I'm still alive is because the spirit wants to live," she said. "It's not really me, anymore. Not the real me, anyway."

She reached for the remote and turned on the TV. We watched an episode of *Law and Order*. "You know why I love this show?" she asked.

"Why?"

"Because I always know how it's going to end. There's no uncertainty. The bad guys get caught."

She was asleep within minutes, and I stayed in the bedroom with her, with my laptop, working away on our book. If I did nothing else, I would finish the book while she was still alive. In every other respect, and especially as a physician, I felt completely helpless. Sometimes, we doctors find it hard to believe that we can't help. We think there must be *something* we can do, and that we're simply not looking hard enough, not thinking clearly enough.

Deb grew progressively weaker. She was often cold and had to be covered with mountains of blankets. And all she ate was a little yogurt with blueberries. Still, she never failed to put on her earrings and a touch of lipstick. "It's not vanity," she told me. "I think it's the least I can do. You're the ones who have to look at me."

A compliment at that point would have been dishonest, and I couldn't be dishonest with her. I could have told her she looked pretty, I imagine, but she was literally withering away. Her face was tired, malnourished; her beauty had faded.

"Let's work on the book," she said.

She was too weak to write, so I set a tape recorder next to the bed. She spoke in bits and starts until she was too exhausted to continue.

"I should get a little sleep," she said. "Two of my friends from the university are stopping by later."

"You need anything else?"

"Ativan would be nice," she said.

I gave her a tablet and she washed it down with water.

"Having you here is very helpful," she said, sighing. "We all appreciate it, especially Giles. My poor Giles. I know he didn't expect it to end this way."

"Are you warm enough?"

"I want you to go through my things and take anything you want," she said.

"I don't want anything," I said. "I just want this wonderful friendship to continue."

"I'm so tired," she said.

I sat with her until she drifted off.

Later that day, her two friends from the university came to visit. Deb reached for her earrings and put on a little lipstick, and we helped her into the living room. She sat on the couch, under a pile of blankets, and I went to get some cheese and crackers.

Deb was laughing and trying hard to look animated, but she was a ghost of her former self. The visitors couldn't hide their fear, or their sorrow. It was clear that they were in awe of Deb, as a human being, as an intellectual, and as a force of nature, but it was equally clear that she wasn't the person she'd been. Still, they got through it. They talked about colleagues and old friends, people I didn't know, until Deb was too exhausted to continue. "It is so nice to see you both, but I'm tired now, and I'm going to need to go back to bed," she said. At that point, as if on cue, both men started to cry. "You know I love you," Deb said. "We always had so much fun."

Giles helped Deb back to her room, and I walked the guests to the front door. Both of them were crushed with grief.

I made my way back upstairs and found Deb still inching her way back to the bedroom, with Giles close at her heels. "Stop hovering!" she snapped at him.

"I'm sorry," Giles said. "The doctor told me to hover, and I'm going to hover."

Deb was a fiercely independent woman, and she hated being so frail and needy—hated the fact that Giles was there to catch her if she fell. But as upset as she was, she still hadn't lost her sense of humor. As they slowly worked their way into the bedroom, she turned to Giles and said, "We need to rethink the terms of our relationship."

Giles laughed and helped her into bed, and I went back downstairs and parked myself in front of my laptop. I stayed up late into the night, transcribing her words.

In the morning, when she was awake, I showed her the pages. She was so tired she could hardly hold them up, but she turned to look at me and laughed her big laugh. "Lois, you rascal, we did it! We really did it!"

"Yes," I said. "We did."

"I want you to promise me one thing."

"Name it."

"If you get on *Oprah*, you'll take Abby with you."

"I promise," I said.

"I'm going to miss you so much," she said.

"Not as much as I'll miss you."

Later that morning, Giles had to go to his office for a short time, and Deb told me she wanted to take a shower.

"Let's wait until Giles gets back, or until the hospice worker gets here," I said.

"No," she said. "I want to take a shower now."

I helped her out of bed and half-carried her into the bathroom. It was all I could do to keep myself from bursting into tears. She was naked and weak and wobbly, and so skinny that her ribs were showing. This was not the way I wanted to remember her.

"Don't fall," I said. "If you fall I am going to be in a lot of trouble."

"I'm not going to fall."

She got the shower started, and I helped her inside, and I kept my hand on her the whole time to steady her. I cried, but I didn't let her see it, and I pulled myself together before she was done.

I helped dry her and got her back into bed.

"I'm out of breath and I haven't even done anything," she said. "Honestly—how long can this go on?"

In the early afternoon, shortly after Giles got back, Congresswoman Lois Capps came to visit.

At one point, Deb reached for pages from our book with great excitement and tried to read. But she couldn't focus and she kept losing her place. "No, wait. Where was I? Here we are!" It was painful to watch, mostly because Deb was aware of her confusion, and her awareness only added to the despair.

Some weeks earlier, she had written about despair—about two episodes in particular. When she was resting, I dug up our book-in-progress and took another look at what she'd said:

I want to say something about the darkness of being a patient. I have had at least two episodes of absolute despair when I was incapable of extracting myself from what John Bunyan so aptly described as the "Slough of Despond." I had entered a realm in which I was incapable of managing my feelings. It followed that I could not control my body, and tears and hysteria had taken me over. The first followed a lovely day at home, spent working on the book. The second was a good deal more public and occurred during a cystogram, where my hysteria, tears, begging, and squirming rendered me an uncooperative patient. Those two experiences—the first occurring by myself and the second in the hospital—hardened my rosy picture of the doctor and/or technician and patient relationship. It was really not so complementary and it requires a good deal of self-discipline on the part of the patient. It requires personal discipline to manage one's illness. The physician can't do it for you. You have to do it. Through these experiences, I realized that the human activity of attentive self-discipline is critical in living through fatal illness. We can all go to the Slough of Despond, but it is easier to get there than to return.

The first episode can best be described as an unraveling. I had an appointment with Dr. Sun at 4:00 P.M. As I began to unravel at 3:00 P.M., the tears and hysteria suggested that I could not dress myself or wash, and the prospect of driving was terrifying. I phoned

Dr. Sun and then called Giles at the university. I am fifty-six and I have seen a lot in the world, but I have never been so completely unstrung. Giles had never seen me that way. And if I said to you that there were certain thoughts that I was thinking, that would be meaningless.

I asked myself if it was fear of death. Maybe. Fear of oblivion? Perhaps. However, the real fear was a fear of despair. And I felt so terrified and I am not sure why. I felt myself going down the hole. I was working on the book, a section that reviewed a part where I was diagnosed with a second cancer. And now I was reading it with a much more fatalistic view. I now clearly had a sense of an ending.

It was a complicated internal exchange. Was some of it also simply missing life itself? Yes, that is really true. I love life. I love the life I have created with Giles. I really do. It has been a great time. And you know what I think constitutes a real life? It is conversation, travel, good food, an intellectual life, and teaching, and the knowledge there is always so much more to know.

And there was something else: After a long conversation with a dear friend from the East, I became overwhelmed with envy—outraged by the unfairness of illness.

How did I get out of it? Ah, Ativan. God bless that stuff. And Giles and Dr. Sun. We had a two-hour conversation with Dr. Sun. "Well," I said, "I don't mind being sick, but I don't like to be in this place, the Slough of Despond, so absolutely without hope."

Dr. Sun said that these experiences would become more frequent, and that I would have to learn to manage myself. There was no way out. It was the nature of illness. There was no running away from it. She also said not to live in the future, not to think about what was coming, but to live each day. I tried to do this, and I am trying still. I stay in the present—painting, talking, sleeping.

The future will take care of itself, I thought, and the past is only something insufficiently remembered.

My second Slough of Despond occurred during a cystogram. I think many of the tests done on people who are terminally ill serve no purpose for the ill. They serve the physician's larger sense of curiosity. Just what is going on here? What is the purpose? They want to know the process. The tests serve no greater good for the patient and often require that the patient sacrifice comfort. If they wanted to help, they would give the patient a pill.

Part of the team that day was a lovely nurse who came in during the cystogram, and I talked to her after she put the long tubing into my bladder. I told her, "I am going to die from what looks like kidney failure, and this test will simply suggest the accuracy of this possibility. What good could this really do any of us?" She looked at me with dear kindness. Then the guys came in, and, holy shit, they just didn't give a damn—they were just going to shoot the dye into the kidney and get this to happen. I said, "It is not happening. It is clogged up." They held me down and tried again, and I felt claustrophobic. I kept wriggling, trying to get out of the way, but they wouldn't talk to me. I was too shaken to yell. I had a sense of violation, but that term may be too easy for a woman to use.

We all left the room with the sense that we had not performed well. No one felt good about it.

. . .

After I finished reading this, overwhelmed, I called Nuri to let him know I missed him. Jessica got on the phone, and I told her I'd be home soon. Then I went back upstairs to see Deb. She was awake but very weak. We looked at each other quietly for a few moments, then she turned her head toward the glass doors. I followed her gaze. A pair of dolphins swam past and we watched them until they were out of sight.

Just then, Abby came into the room. "Mom," she said. "Can I borrow a pair of socks?"

"You can borrow them," Deb said, and she smiled. "But I'm not gone yet."

Abby laughed. So did I. It was nice to see that Deb hadn't lost her sense of humor. Abby had already moved back home from the university over a month before to help care for her mom, as she had done on weekend and vacation visits during and long before her college years.

Abby took the socks, but she paused by the bed, looked at her mother, then turned to me and studied my growing belly. She put her hand on it, and Deb reached over and did the same. They waited like that for a few moments, hoping for a kick.

"She must be sleeping," I said.

After Abby left, Deb told me that some weeks earlier, when she still had a little strength, she'd gone to visit some old friends. "I was pushing myself," she said. "I was trying to live or at least to act alive, but it was a very disappointing experience."

"How so?"

"These women were sitting around talking about 'life lessons' and what not, and they kept looking over at me, as if I, the Dying Friend, was just brimming over with wisdom—as if I had all the answers."

She was angry. At the women, for wanting answers, and at life—for not providing them.

"When you ask a Jewish person what heaven is, they throw up their hands and say, 'Who knows?! And why should I worry about it?' Well, that's my answer. I don't know and I'm not going to worry about it." She took a moment and seemed to reconsider. "But it would be great if I could come back."

She once told me that she liked being Jewish, but that she wasn't *particularly* Jewish. Still, it was part of her identity. She may have wanted to be a Christian at that moment, may have wanted to believe that St. Peter really was waiting for her at the Gates of Heaven, and she may have wanted to be a Buddhist, wanted to know in her heart that she was really coming back, and that—thanks to her good karma —her new life would be a pleasant surprise. But, alas, she could only be who she was, and she was —as she'd told Abby—*a Jewish white girl*.

I went home the following day, but two weeks later she took another turn for the worse, and I returned to Santa Barbara.

Giles was waiting for me at the house. He looked drawn and tired and very sad, and he drove me to the hospital.

When we walked into her room, she was as small and weak as I'd ever seen her, but she looked up and managed a small smile.

"We're going to take you home," Giles said.

We got her home and got her situated in her bedroom. She studied the ocean from her king-sized bed. The waves rolled in, crashing against the giant rocks near shore.

Later that day, a nurse stopped by the house to show her how to feed the antibiotics though the IV. When she left, Deb and I found ourselves alone. "I'm not happy about this so-called *prospect of departure,*" she said.

"What can I do to help?"

"I don't know. I'm not really in pain, but I feel like I can't breathe very well."

"Use the oxygen," I said.

"Do you think I need it?"

"Yes. There's no harm in using the oxygen."

I helped her with the oxygen. She took a few deep breaths and seemed to relax a little. The sun was just beginning to set.

"You know, Lois, this time I think I'm really done," she said. "Let's talk about the stash."

"What have you got squirreled away?"

She reached into the drawer next to her bed and pulled out a wrinkled, brown paper bag. There were three bottles inside: potassium tablets, Oxycontin, and morphine. She held them aloft and looked to me for advice.

"I really don't know," I said. "You'd probably throw up before you could get many of them down, so it might only make things worse."

"I don't want to live like this," she said. "I can't eat. I can't talk. And even when I enjoy the company of friends, I don't enjoy it."

I didn't say anything.

"Should I stop the antibiotics?" she asked.

I looked at her. Sometimes a patient needs permission to stop treatment, particularly if they think it's futile, and that seemed to be what Deb was doing. "The antibiotics are designed to ward off infection," I said. "If you stop taking them, there's a good chance that will work more effectively than your little stash."

"So that would end it?"

"Probably."

"I hear pneumonia is an old person's friend," she said.

"It's one way to die," I said.

Giles walked in and heard the last part of this conversation. "You're going to need to share this decision with your children," he said, and he left the room to get them.

Deb looked at me. "It's just too hard," she said.

"I know," I replied.

Giles returned a short time later, with Abby and Adam. Giles knelt by the side of the bed. I looked at him, wondering if I should leave, but he shook his head no he wanted me there. He took Deb's hand and told her he loved her. Adam stood by the foot of the bed, quiet, unmoving, and Abby curled up next to her mother and began stroking her hair.

"I've thought about this," Deb said. "And I'm really done this time."

She glanced over at me, then looked back at her family. "I know I've said it before, but this time I mean it. I've really had enough."

Abby bit her lip, crying. "If that's what you want, Mom," she said. "I understand."

I remember marveling at how this girl, who had spent her entire adolescence terrified, like so many others in her situation, that her mother might die, nonetheless remained throughout such a fiercely loyal and loving daughter. The years were difficult, but here was the teenager who had become a young woman by never letting go of that thirst for life she shared so intimately with her mom.

"That's what I want."

"Is there any way you can stick around?" Abby asked.

Deb smiled at her. "If I can, I will," she said.

"I want to say something else, Mom."

"Go ahead, honey."

"I want to thank you for being my mom, and for fighting so hard to stay in this world to help me grow up. It has been an honor and a privilege to be your daughter. If there's any way I can make your leaving easier, let me know and I'll do it."

By this time all of us were crying. I couldn't help thinking about how amazing this mother-daughter relationship had become and how much joy Abby's words had given Deb.

As a result of such transparent honesty and intimacy, we all slept slightly better that night, knowing that love can sometimes bring peace to even the most anguished hearts. The next day, the nurse arrived to administer the antibiotics, and Deb told her she didn't want them—that she had decided to discontinue all treatment. The nurse remained spirited and confident, inspired by her mission to help, but after assessing the situation she asked Deb what she imagined would happen after the end of her life.

Deb shared her previous experience during bone marrow transplantation and of coming so close to death. She told the nurse of the unity she felt with all nature, implying she expected the same when she died. It was so beautiful, so universal. She reflected on the words of Psalm 40 . . . *all flesh is grass* . . . and spoke about becoming part of a larger whole.

The nurse seemed to change gears here, and she began to talk about her own experiences in loving, and being loved by, God. This was very unprofessional and unsettling, and in many ways transgressed the integrity, even the *sanctity*, of the relationship between the health-care giver and the patient. Most caregivers know it is so important to "go where the patient is," to be with them and support their beneficial coping methods and belief systems. Instead, she went on and on about her own life, and how it had been transformed by faith, saying that God's undying love for every living being was the one thing that really mattered.

"It breaks my heart to imagine people dying and not having met the love and power of Jesus Christ," she said.

The conversation, which had been personal and yet completely universal at the same time, was over, a dialogue replaced by monologue. The beauty of what Deb had said had been completely discounted, a delicate understanding sullied by a more narrow view, and suddenly I perceived a wall separating us from the nurse. Fortunately, as a result of sincerity and good intentions, the conversation continued civilly, but only because Deb never took the bait—only because Deb was too exhausted and could not allow herself to be angry. But I was disappointed and Giles was angry and felt like wringing her neck. This was exactly the wrong thing to say to anyone in such extremity—much less to Deb—much less to a Jewish professor of the history of world religions!

Facing the end of life is interesting because I have already experienced it with the bone marrow transplant, which is a simulation of dying. It is an experience in which you lose your life principle, your life energy. And as all that closes down—and it does—you have to go way inside, deep inside, and you are maintained in life by other means: by other people's platelets, by antibiotics, by blood. Then if it works, those little Debs find their way back to the stem cells, and they reawaken you.

It is not personal. It is the same creative energy that makes the grass green. You could be the grass, a fish, a frog—it is all part of the same thing. When it takes form in me, it becomes Deb cells, but that's not going to last for very long.

I really felt that I was part of the universe. So why worry? There was a larger sense of unity with all the forces of the cosmos, and the form "Deb" had taken was impermanent and open for revision.

Do I imagine that I will meet up with the beloved dead when I join their society? I would love to run into Giles. I would love

*to be with Giles and Abby and Adam—and Brahms—but who
knows if I am going to run into them? I might run into them later,
but I will know later, maybe. And, of course, I would like to come
back here to my home overlooking the ocean; who wouldn't?*

I don't think we need to go with Jesus.

In the course of the next two days, a steady parade of people
came by the house to see Deb. Friends, colleagues, students,
neighbors.

Tired as she was, Deb never failed to put on her earrings
and her lipstick. The conversations were brief, and usually
exhausting, and at one point even the sound of the tearful
farewells was more than she could bear. Afer the third such
visit, which was as searing as it was loving, Deb looked over at
Giles and suggested, "Why don't we change 'goodbye' to 'see
you later'?"

Abby's friends came, too, as did Adam's fiancée, DeAnn,
and at one point the house was bustling with so much energy
that it seemed to lift Deb's spirits. She even began to eat well,
which prompted Giles to joke with me, "She always eats when
you're around!"

"Yes," I said. "It's one of the many things we did well
together!"

The pain persisted, however, growing worse, and Deb
took larger and larger doses of liquid morphine. She slept
often, and she needed help moving about, and I found myself
thinking again—selfishly, misguidedly—that there must be

other treatments we had overlooked. There weren't, of course. I simply wasn't ready to let her go.

Adam didn't want to let go, either. He had had a difficult history with Deb, especially during his teenaged years, as often happens when a parent remarries, but from the beginning of her illness he had become a steady presence and a solid source of support, and the family had come to rely on him. He was a good listener, and he was always the first to volunteer when something needed doing. One night, Deb turned to him and said, "One of the great accomplishments of my life, as well as one of its great joys, is the fact that you call me 'Mom.'"

I shared my love for Deb with her family. I was there for five days, and I told them stories about some of the things we'd shared. *The Lion King. Carmen.* The Eiffel Tower. The warm marble slabs at that spa in Turkey. The memorable meals. The many, many shopping expeditions.

"What's the big deal?" she had said. "It's not like I'm planning for retirement."

It was the first time in a long time I had seen them laughing.

At one point I found myself alone with Abby, and we held each other. "I love your mother so much," I told her. "I'm going to miss everything about her."

"Especially her laugh," Abby said.

"Yes. Especially her laugh."

"'Ya think?'" Abby said, mimicking Deb perfectly, but a moment later she was sobbing.

"Your mother made the world a richer, better place for

me," I said. "I don't know how to say goodbye to her. I don't want to say goodbye."

Later that day, I packed my bag and braced myself and went into her room. "Deb," I said. "I have to go now. I've got to get back to Houston." I sat on the edge of her bed and hugged her and held her close, but I didn't cry. And I didn't say goodbye. I just couldn't do it.

"Oh, Lois," she said. "I love you. I will miss you and the fun we had together. I want you to go home, love your husband, love your children, and live a big life."

I was crying by the time I got into my rented car, and I cried all the way to the airport. I called Nuri en route, sobbing, and I called my mother, still sobbing.

When I got back to Houston, I wrote Deb a letter, and I cried through every word and beyond:

March 29, 2006

Dear Deb,

I don't think I could say goodbye without really losing it and I don't want to think this is the last time I am going to talk to you. I will just try to fit some of what I want to say in the next few paragraphs.

I just want you to know how much I cherish and treasure the person you are and how special I feel to be such a close friend. You have made my life so much richer. The special conversations, visits, travel, food, experiences and your time have meant so much to me. This world will not be the same without you, but knowing you has made it a far better place for me. I love your style, your charm, your creativity, your smile and I especially love your laugh. Actually I envy your laugh and the hardiness with which it explodes out of your "deep inside." I can only hope to have the experiences you have had, the loves you have loved, and the friends who love you so much. I too will try to live in the present moment—not worrying about what may or may not come, especially as we really don't know.

I also want to tell you, again, how much it meant to me and Nuri that you spoke at our wedding. What you said was so beautiful. My family loves you and knowing you are in the world has affected them deeply, also.

I will miss your visits—both you and Giles. I plan and need to keep in touch with your wonderful family as much as I can, not just to help, but to grow our friendships even stronger and to keep the connection to you. I hope they want to do the same. I see Abby as this wonderful creative person—very different from you but still with enough similarity that I can smile at the Deb that lives inside her. I can't wait to know her more over the years. I plan to watch her, know her, and be available to her for years to come. (I hope she will remember me when she is famous!)

I realized yesterday that the book has been a way to make sure I never forget a minute of the times we have spent together. I will forever treasure this timeless form in which our friendship will live. It is interesting that today I really did understand that the reason for writing was not to document my medical life or your cancer life. Nor was the book written to further either of our careers. In fact, it was part of the friendship, part of what we did together, a good reason to get together—a unique experience that is really not accessible to many friends. Think of the times we wrote: Le Grand Colbert, the cafes in Paris, the Bebek, your beautiful backyard, my old kitchen table, my new home. . . . We have become better, closer, and more sincere (naked?) friends as a result of the book. Our friendship evolved partially through the writing. More so, it has furthered my understanding of my self and you through our reflections of each other. It is a celebration of our friendship, and I'm already having trouble imagining how I'm going to celebrate without you. I wish we could have written in Marrakech, Milan, Madrid. I know you too would have gotten so much joy out of living that experience. Part of me continues to hope for a miracle—one that gives you improved function and energy and time.

I wish you peace of mind and an end to pain and suffering. These last few days have been so beautiful for me to be part of and I thank you so much for taking me in as part of your Gunn-Sills family. It is an honor which is indescribable and one I will never forget. I hope I have helped although I am not sure how I did. I wish I could stay and be a part of every last day. I can't wait to tell Leila Rose Nuri all about you. I wish I never had to say goodbye so I will call you soon. I can only hope that you will have the energy to talk with me for much time to come.

I love you so much—my life will be lacking without you in it.

Lois

I called Deb every two or three days, but she was weak and could never talk for very long.

At the time, Jessie and I were reading a book called *The Fall of Freddie the Leaf*, by Leo Buscaglia. It's a story about a little leaf that begins to understand the passage of time, and eventually comes to terms with the inevitability of death, and I was reading it more for me than for Jessica. I found it very comforting.

Sometimes, after Jessica was asleep, I'd read Nuri passages from our own book, this work-in-progress, and it made Deb come alive for me again, took me back to better days. There had been times along the way when I wondered if we'd become *too* close, but I realized it hadn't been a choice. Our friendship simply happened, and it was one of the great blessings of my life.

Making my rounds in the hospitals during this period, I stopped saying goodbye to my dying patients. Instead, I would say, "Call me anytime." Or, "See you." Or, "You are in my thoughts."

Goodbye had such finality. I still hadn't said goodbye to Deb, and I didn't think I ever would.

On April 30, 2006, Nuri and I celebrated our one-year anniversary. I called Deb to talk to her, but she was on morphine and not terribly coherent, and she had been moved back to the hospital to help her manage the pain. I told her that I was thinking of her, and that I loved her, and then I went off to get ready for our guests. We had an open house. People came by to eat and to celebrate, and many of them took the time to pat my swollen belly. The party went very late, and Nuri and I cleaned up a little before dropping into bed, exhausted.

The phone woke us early the next morning. It was Giles. He was crying. "Deb's gone," he said.

I flew out for the funeral. Nuri and Jessica came with me. Hundreds of people turned out, and many of them shared memories of Deb. I read a brief excerpt from our book, the section that began *"All I wanted to do after my initial diagnosis with ovarian cancer was to dance . . .*

"I had danced casually as a kid and a teenager, but it was my mother's drunken afternoons that derailed my afternoon trips to Brown Gables Academy of Dance, in Los Angeles. I didn't drive and she didn't want to. Yet ballet has always been alive in a distant place in my imagination.

"I danced through college and then, with a great deal of commitment, through graduate school . . . I became a sort of middle-aged mascot to the professional ballet company in Santa Barbara. I couldn't do the pliés and pirouettes that were once part of my repertoire, but I was alive . . .

So many people came, even Dr. Bouquet came from Houston, their relationship, like Deb's with so many of the people who treated her, was quickly to turn into something very special when she and Dr. Bouquet discovered that they shared not only a desire to address her disease but a passionate interest in history and ideas.

Other people spoke. They described Deb as eccentric, brilliant, passionate, charismatic. They talked about her style, and her grace, and about the energy that seemed to lift everyone that stepped into her circle. And they talked about her laugh. God, how I miss that laugh!

As I stood there, crying, I remembered our lunch at that café in Paris, and the woman at the neighboring table who had stopped by on her way out. "Excuse me," she had told Deb. "I have been watching you, and I must say: There's a powerful light coming from inside of you!"

Leila Rose Nuri was born on June 8, 2006. Sometimes, when she looks at me, I can see Deb in her eyes—I can see the same light shining inside her.

AFTERWORD

by Giles Gunn

Deborah died on the first of May 2006, to the strains of Mozart's *Requiem*. Adam had set up a recorder, which allowed all of Deborah's favorite Mozart music to play continuously over the three days and nights we spent with her in the hospital. At a certain point it had become too difficult to manage the increasing pain at home, despite the only intermittently successful service of a hospice group, and so she consented, at Dr. Sun's suggestion and with our support, to being moved.

The end was not as any of us had—or could have—imagined it. We knew that we would all be together in this moment, but we never quite realized—who can?—how precious and agonizing it would be. Deborah soon went into a deep sleep but twice came out of it full of expectation and radiance to greet the arrival of a dear friend from Paris and then, the next day, a rabbi friend. Both awakenings felt like a miracle, even if unbearably fleeting, but the real act of transcendence—more like translucence—occurred the night before and then the night (really early morning) of her passing.

I had been lying with her in the hospital bed when, from across a divide that already seemed impassable, she began to sigh. And when I spoke, and then later Abby and Adam, she would respond to our words but in ways, almost inaudible ways, that surpassed a simple recognition of our presence. We were actually, unbelievably, conversing in a medium of purest desire, on the first night on and off for several hours, on the second for a much shorter time. She was communicating with us merely through the most fragile exhalations of breath, but we felt bathed in something as close to the source of conscious life as human beings may be able to experience. We talked of our love mostly, and of the children, and of our desire for her suffering to cease, and of the unbearable difficulties of parting. And then she was gone.

Throughout this process, Dr. Sun was almost continuously present or available even if she was seeing other patients. And the nurses on Deb's floor were angelic in their mercy and kindness. Dying can be a difficult, even harrowing, or sometimes simple art, but rarely, I have come to appreciate, is it attended by professionals who care so much about seeing to it, as Deborah so much wanted, that it is done well. This took inconceivable grit on Deborah's part and produced inconsolable loss on ours. But again, Deborah deserved the last word: While you may not ever get over it, she used to say, you still need to get on with it. And so we began.

Deborah did not want a service but merely a party where the things she so much loved, friendship, good food, interesting conversation, laughter, could commingle in her honor. Abby, Adam, and I agreed with the last part of this plan but had to override her wishes on the first. We would have a ceremony to commemorate her passing, but include within it an invitation to join us for lunch and beyond at a party to celebrate her life. Thanks to those who spoke—among them Dr. Lois, seven months pregnant, who returned for the third time in five weeks, this time with Nuri and their daughter, Jessica; Dr. Sun, Deb's oncologist whose solidarity over the years was as equally remarkable as her skill; Congresswoman Lois Capps, whose family was so much a part of ours and in whose house we were married; devoted colleagues from California Lutheran University (who represented part of her wonderful, special support group on campus); and, most movingly and bravely, Abby—together with the music and many family members and friends from all parts of Deborah's past, including Dr. Robert Bouquet and his wife, dearest of friends from M. D. Anderson, the memorial service took on a radiance that was almost palpable, and the party later took care of itself.

Adam's marriage to DeAnn occurred a month later. It was a small ceremony in a beautiful place, with the bride's parents joining Abby, me, and one of my college roommates, who conducted the ceremony. Deborah was also in her way vividly present, most especially when Abby read words from a wedding blessing that Deborah had originally prepared for Dr. Lois and Nuri's ceremony and then adapted to Adam and

DeAnn's. The words, drawn from the Preacher of Ecclesiastes, speak of life as being better with two rather than one, because if one falls, the other will lift his fellow, just as two lying together is better than one, for how, the Preacher asks, can one be warm alone? Deborah also believed with the philosopher Stanley Cavell—and stated in her comments to Adam and DeAnn—that all happy marriages are really re-marriages. Good marriages, in other words, are always in the process of re-creating and revising, restoring, if you will, the original marriage, but often on altered or different footing. She also referred to marriage as a kind of Balanchine pas de deux, a conversation between two adults whose continuing happiness results in part from never quite knowing what the other will say.

Adam's wedding was followed two weeks later by Abby's graduation. This was an event that Deborah would have been willing to give her heart's last breath to attend, but that breath had already done its work. Abby had always known of the boundless joy her mother took in her accomplishments, often against difficult odds, and she now lived with the knowledge we had all taken away from the hospital room in those early morning hours on May 1 when Deborah gave us her blessing to live beyond her. Had Deborah somehow survived long enough to attend Abby's graduation, she would have been hallelujahing and stomping even from a wheelchair, but we got through the ceremony without her actual presence because we knew that she was still so much a part of it, and of us.

The last episode of this story belongs to the actual birth of

Leila Rose Nuri on June 8. This was the event toward which, as Deborah and Dr. Lois came to understand, their narrative was ultimately pointed. If Deborah's life didn't last long enough to reach that goal, the story of her relationship with Dr. Lois nonetheless found its consummation there, at least for the moment. After all, this is a story about wresting new life from mortal instruments. But new life, as most cancer patients and their caregivers know, is not to be confused with physical health; it is rather to be identified with the courage to extract the wisdom from the hardest things. Deborah was, and with Dr. Lois's marvelous collaboration, remains, a teacher who possessed the gifts to turn all living into a form of learning, all learning into a kind of art enhanced, wherever possible, with style, humor, wit, beauty, and courage.

APPENDIX

THE INTERVIEW

Abby: All right, and we are discussing death, and you are someone who has come up against . . .

Deb: Many times! (Laughs.)

Abby: Could you please explain your . . . ?

Deb: I was diagnosed with ovarian, Stage III ovarian cancer when I was um, my God, forty-eight, six years ago and um, I have been in chemotherapy virtually, surgeries and so forth, ever since.

Abby: Yes, and in particular you had a bone marrow transplant?

Deb: Oh, uh, big time. So I did have the experience of dying and rising again.

Abby: And uh, in that experience, there was something you said to me which was—do you remember when you talked about the ummm, the actual . . . ?

Deb: Oh, oh yes.

Abby: . . . dying and coming back.

Deb: You want me to uh, do that? That's a good one.

Abby: That's a good one.

Deb: Well, the bone marrow transplant—a project of a bone marrow transplant is to take out bone marrow before they give you so much chemotherapy that they virtually kill you, that is, they kill your body's ability to maintain itself in life. So, for a period that can range from eight days to two weeks you're in a kind of limbo where you are literally, uh, actually I should say, maintained in life by other means; that is by people's, uh, platelets, blood, lots of antibiotics, and you do, I did, have this experience of dying, that is all my systems were shutting down. . . . couldn't hear very well, couldn't see, couldn't read very well, was real angry. After the chemotherapy which lasts a week— God, I can't even imagine we did that—they give you back the stem cells and you wait for something to happen.

And it's interesting, I felt it long before the doctors told me my blood counts had started to rise. And I felt it in my dreams, and I felt it in the music I wanted to listen to, and what I felt was—I have to use the language of a dear friend of mine who is now dead, Louis Netzer, but he used to quote the French philosopher, Henri Bergson, who would talk about the "élan vital," the sort of—the vitality that is part of life. And Buddhists would talk about it, or Hindus perhaps, as a kind of spiritual component, or the thing that enlivens matter, but in any event it was leaving me, or had left me to a considerable degree, and then

I felt it come back to life. And probably the most striking thing about it was that it wasn't personal, [. . .] that I had the distinct impression that what was returning to me was the stuff that made the grass green, made kids laugh, and it was the thing that enlivened the world—and it wasn't personal. It took personal form when it was in me, but in itself, it was not personal, it was a kind of life force. How's that?

Abby: Perfect.

Deb: That's good?

Abby: Yeah. So in that experience, after that experience, do you now fear death in the way that you used to? . . . Because, I mean I don't know, did you used to fear death when you were first diagnosed?

Deb: Oh yeah! Well, I still don't want to die.

Abby: Right, but do you fear the actual . . .

Deb: The passage?

Abby: Yeah.

Deb: I'm hoping to have enough drugs so that I won't feel it too considerably. But yeah, I do. Well, I don't. I mean, I would say—and I've seen this in people, in the world of cancer treatment—that there's a time to go.

Abby: Uh-huh.

Deb: I saw that with [my friend] Louis. That is, he just—life had become too difficult, it had become too difficult to live because his body had given out on him. Saw that in Lisa Capps.

Abby: Yeah.

Deb: And I'm sure we'll see it in me. At some point.

Abby: Yeah.

Deb: Um, and then that transition, I don't know, it's a different thing to say about are you afraid of it . . . What I want now is to wring out of life everything I can before I hit that wall.

Abby: But okay, let's go back to the beginning when all of this started and you were first diagnosed. Do you feel like the way that you were raised, or your family's approach to death . . . Did your family even talk about death?

Deb: Well, we had a death early on, when I was five years old, my parents . . . I mean it's a terrible story . . .

Abby: You can go into it a little bit.

Deb: All right, ummm, my parents had a terr— They had a second child when I was just five and this baby was eight days old, given a prescription for colic, went into shock, and died six hours later. Uh, and that, I mean, that's bad. But then what made it truly horrible was that the police then accused my father of poisoning the baby, so we had this horrific experience of, not only death, but the state, punishment, victimization, all of that. And we all tried to ignore it as best we could, but it was very public—it went to court.

Abby: Did they actually try your dad?

Deb: No no no. After six months, they investigated him and [my mother] Dolly . . . I remember going to the police station and sitting in the police station with Dolly, waiting for her to be questioned. Their tactic, something out of *Law and Order,* was to go after what they thought was the weak link, that is, the mother, and then she would turn and give evidence on Irvin. The police called her every single day, and at one point she stopped answering the phone, and Irvin drove home in a fury, sure that she had hanged herself in the garage. I mean, it was a bad business.

Abby: Yeah. A very bad business.

Deb: Bad business. That and then, you know, when the second child was born, the brother who survived, he became mortally ill as a teenager, but survived. [. . .]

Abby: And would you say that with cancer, as opposed to— because you've said this before, that a good death is a quick one. You don't know it's coming and it's just, boom! As opposed to a prolonged. . . .

Deb: Well, you know, I've said that but I don't know that it's true. I mean, the stuff I've read about, you know—people are frightened to die. But I think when you get right up to it . . . I don't know. I'll let you know . . .

Abby: Right.

Deb: But people say, "Oh, I'm not the first person to die. I bet I can do it!" (Laughs.) "I bet I can do it!" And it's funny, when I think about [my friend] Walter [Capps] dying, you know, he had this massive heart attack. And there's part of me that thinks his heart burst because he was having so much fun. You know? He was just overwhelmed. He liked being a congressman so much, and he looked fabulous. . . .

Abby: He really did.

Deb: He just looked fabulous. At the same time, I would say that my experience of looking at the finite character of life has made me a more interesting teacher. It has probably made me a better mother, too.

Abby: Yeah.

Deb: That is, I realize that mothering is not about my life; it is about my kid's life. And at this point, what I would say is that unlike [my friend] Lisa, you know, who died when her kids were a year and a half and six years old. . . .

Abby: Yeah?

Deb: You know, it scared me when you were thirteen, and I was diagnosed, I thought—and in fact I remember Dr. Darling, when I first interviewed her, or she interviewed me, about the bone marrow transplant, I remember saying, "I have to stay in the world because I have a young teenage daughter and she's not ready for me to go yet." But now I would say now, "My daughter is in college. She would love to have me in the world, but I look at her and I say to myself, You know, she's okay. She can live on her own. She can make judgments about herself and be okay. She can manage it." But when you were thirteen or even sixteen I was much too frightened for you.

Abby: Yeah, because your family was in crisis after your diagnosis.

Deb: Ohhh, I think probably every family goes into crisis when you face this. Absolutely.

Abby: Why?

Deb: Because we live with the myth that children are supposed to bury their parents. And because death is hard.

Abby: What do you mean by the myth? You've said before
that if all goes right, children do bury their parents, and
that's true. But you know, when you read the obituaries
and you see like an eighty-five—

Deb: (Laughs.)

Abby: Okay. I read the obituaries . . .

Deb: I do, too.

Abby: Well, you know, and you see, you see . . . an eighty-
four-year-old woman dead, it's okay, but when they're
fifty-two—

Deb: Then you probably think they're leaving kids who are
about your age.

Abby: It's not even that. It's like a sense of things not being
done, not finished. And I wonder, you know, because
you've been fighting this for almost seven years now,
which is . . . Wait, isn't, aren't you, you're—you're in, like,
the seventeenth percentile of people who make it this far?

Deb: You bet.

Abby: You go! You go with your bad self!

Deb: (laughs)

Abby: But do you think that, since you've had this time, you've
been able to reassess life in a different way? Like you've
made changes so you appreciate it—

Deb: Sure.

Abby: You get to do it on your terms instead of—

Deb: Yeah, but in a way, and I've said this . . . What cancer does for those who are able to manage, if it doesn't kill them immediately, is you're able to look at life as it really is. It's finite. You don't have all the time in the world. And what cancer simply does is remind you of that.

Abby: Uh-huh.

Deb: And so it makes you face it in a way that people who, in effect, haven't faced a mortal illness seldom face it. You can't ignore it.

Abby: But that's—

Deb: And so it's true. The thing is, you know, I've had all the children I'm going to have; I had the good fortune to marry the right guy; I've had this transition into realizing that I really did get to do the work I like to do. And you know, when I first got diagnosed, I thought, "Oh my . . . I can't go back to teaching."

Abby: You were very angry?

Deb: You bet. Wouldn't you have been?

Abby: Oh?

Deb: Pissed off.

Abby: But why—why were you angry?

Deb: Well, I think it's the classic female posture, which is, you know, the joke is "Pardon me, Alphonse." That is, you know, *What can I do for you?* That's the female argument.

Abby: Yeah?

Deb: "What can I do for my husband?" "What can I do for my kids?" And there I was, forty-eight years old, and, shit, maybe I'd put off the things I wanted to do . . .

Abby: Yeah?

Deb: And now I wasn't going to have any time to do it!

Abby: But then, also, I mean, in your life taking care of an alcoholic mother and—

Deb: Sure. All of that stuff.

Abby: You had been a caregiver.

Deb: Yes, but I'm cleaning that up.

Abby: You are?

Deb: It's hooray for me and to hell with you. (Laughs.) Though not you specifically . . .

Abby: No, yes, I realize . . . (Laughs.)

Abby: Yup.

Deb: And as far as the symptoms for ovarian cancer—

Abby: It's like the flu, isn't it?

Deb: Well, you've got bloating, but I've got colitis, so I thought all those symptoms were colitis-related, not ovarian-cancer-related.

Abby: Okay, um, well, let's go back to dying.

Deb: Okay. (Laughs.)

Abby: Is that all right? It's for class—I need to know . . .

Deb: Absolutely.

Abby: You're a historian of religion; you've come across many different kinds of deaths . . .

Deb: Stories about death.

Abby: Exactly. And the afterlife and all that stuff . . .

Deb: Yeah.

Abby: Is there any one that particularly agrees with you, or that has helped you through this process? Or do you sort of believe it's all kind of crap?

Deb: Oh, I wouldn't say that. I'd say that the one that has sort of helped me is, perhaps, well the idea that I get to see Walter, right? And my parents, right?

Abby: Yeah.

Deb: People who have gone, people I was very keen on but who are now dead. That would be a kind of Western model of the afterlife.

Abby: Right.

Deb: You get to meet up with people. But at the same time I like the idea of being able to lay your burden down, a sort of merging with the great oceanic—

Abby: Buddhism?

Deb: Yeah. So I'd say that those two ways of looking at things have helped, and it sort of depends on what I'm in the mood for.

Abby: Okay. And how do you control your death anxiety?

Deb: Through drugs. (Laughs.) Through drugs. Through exercise. Through fun.

Abby: Uh-huh.

Deb: I started taking an antidepressant, and an antianxiety drug, when my husband and my daughter demanded I do it. (Laughs.) And in fact, you know, once I did, I thought, "God, this is a better way to live!" Now I recommend it. I recommend it to everyone.

Abby: Uh-huh.

Deb: Drugs and exercise. And in effect, I haven't had a horrific scare, it's just been incremental. [. . .]

Abby: Would you prefer to have control over the end or to just let it come?

Deb: Well, you know, these are things I have thought about. I have a dear friend, Fran, who is also an ovarian cancer patient, and her disease is probably farther along than mine—though I don't know if that's really the case. Let's say it's less manageable than mine has been. And we talk about it, you know, "Can we lay in a supply of Seconal so that we have that option?" And we've both probably thought about this, and we *don't* have a supply of Seconal (laughs), which may be problematic, but we've thought that—even if we didn't use it—it would be nice to know it was available. In the same way, I was talking to Chantal about Louis. He wanted to have enough narcotics to kill himself, but the interesting thing is that he never used them. He held on until the bitter end. And I think it was very difficult, at the end, because a friend told me that his cancer, bile-duct cancer, produces little pain but a lot of toxicity, and he lost his mind. That's a pisser.

Abby: That's a pisser.

Deb: So, I don't know. I've told you my fantasy of flying to Paris, checking into the Ritz, going to the ballet, and then the restaurant, Le Grand Colbert, then going back to the Ritz and having them find me the next morning. (Laughs.)

Abby: Well, that's technically part of the next question I wanted to ask. (Laughs.) What would be a good death?

Deb: I mean, realistically, one that is not painful, one that is not full of anxiety. Keb' Mo' has this great song where he talks about death as a new beginning. So, philosophically, if it's realistic, I would like not to be afraid . . .

Abby: Uh-huh.

Deb: I'd like to not hurt, and I'd like not to be too pissed off. But you know, the interesting thing I would say is, I mean, it's quite remarkable—nobody wants to die. I mean, I [knew] an eighty-something woman who'd been diagnosed with ovarian, late Stage III, and she had surgery and did chemotherapy and went to an aerobics class and looked at herself in the mirror and said, "My God! I look like a ninety-year-old woman!" (Laughs.) Nobody wants to go. The fact that I don't want to go at fifty-four doesn't mean I'd want to go at sixty. I still wouldn't want to go. But I think with cancer when you're ready, when it's time to die, it's because your body has given out on you to such a degree that you're just hoping you can just relax and let go.

Abby: That sounds . . .

Deb: God. Can I say one thing?

Abby: Please, please.

Deb: One of the reasons I don't want to die, a big reason to stay around, is I want to see what my kids do, how they turn out.

Abby: I think your kids . . .

Deb: I want to see what, particularly, my daughter is going to be. She's such an interesting person. And I want to find out what she's going to do. It'd be fun to hang out with her, though not all the time—I promise! (Laughs.) [. . .] But it's a trade-off.

Abby: Well, is it? Because I interviewed a young woman in class, about death, and her reason for being afraid of death was that she didn't want anybody else to hurt—she didn't want anybody else to miss her. So it wasn't exactly the crossing or the passage, if you will, but—

Deb: Is this person sick?

Abby: No.

Deb: That is such a bullshit line! (Laughs.)

Abby: Mom! (Laughs.)

Deb: I mean, it is such a girlish line. "I'm here to serve!"

Abby: Yeah . . .

Deb: "I'm here to make other people's lives better!" God forbid anyone else should hurt. It's a bullshit line. Because when you come right up to it, you're afraid of dying not because of anyone else. You don't want to die 'cause you don't want to leave!

Abby: Yeah, well.

Deb: So she's full of malarkey.

Abby: Do you think you would have said that if you hadn't gotten ill? That same sort of line? "I can't leave. I can't leave my husband. I can't leave my kids."

Deb: Well, you could say that part of me, when I went for the BMT, was because I couldn't leave my daughter.

Abby: That's different.

Deb: But this is a girl—this is a girl in your class. Is she a woman with children?

Abby: No.

Deb: So she's making it up.

Abby: True.

Deb: She's making it all up. And she, she didn't talk to you straight. She talked to you about the role; she gave you a kind of standard female role response.

Abby: So do you believe that there are certain ways we respond—that men aren't supposed to cry, for example?

Deb: I don't know. But in a way, this girl you interviewed, she was not willing to talk about her own pain. She wanted to talk about everybody else's pain.

Abby: [. . .] You've gone to a lot of funerals. Are people supposed to really just bawl?

Deb: Well, it depends.

Abby: When you give the eulogies, though, you're not supposed to bawl, don't you remember Walter's funeral? Everyone was very—maybe because they're Swedish or whatever . . .

Deb: Swedish, yes. (Laughs.) But Jesse Jackson was there, and he said, "Let's clap for Walter."

Abby: I was thinking about this, you know, because I'm sure you've thought about what you want your funeral to be like.

Deb: Isn't that interesting . . .

Abby: You never . . . ?

Deb: I don't give a shit.

Abby: Really?

Deb: No. I'm going to be gone.

Abby: I know, but you don't think, because I once read this article about this young girl who died of, you know, with AIDS, and she planned her entire funeral. It was a celebration. And I was thinking, you know, there's no one right way to deal with death . . .

Deb: You're right.

Abby: And there's no one right way to have a funeral. Why do we have to have flowers, why do you have to have hymns?

Deb: Well, those are Christian funerals.

Abby: What do they do at Jewish funerals?

Deb: Get 'em in the ground real quick. (Laughs.)

Abby: You want to be cremated though, don't you?

Deb: Yeah, but, you know, it's an interesting business. My husband's mother planned her funeral.

Abby: She did?

Deb: Yeah.

Abby: Which one?

Deb: Ooch. Grandma Ooch. She planned her funeral.

Abby: Was it nice? (Laughs.)

Deb: Well, you were there. You just don't remember.

Abby: I was like three.

Deb: Yeah. This is all very interesting. Maybe I haven't faced the details of death yet, but I don't give a shit what you do. I'm going to be gone. So, you know, you know what music I like . . .

Abby: Disco. (Laughs.)

Deb: If you wanted to do disco, or if you wanted to do, you know, Mozart or *Don Giovanni*—

Abby: *Carmina Burana*. I'm kidding, I'm kidding.

Deb: Yeah, would I want *Carmina Burana*?

Abby: No.

Deb: No. But you know, in a way, the funeral is not about the person who died—it's for the people who are left.

Abby: Yeah.

Deb: So maybe it's a good thing that the person who's on their way out tells the person . . .

Abby: Maybe . . .

Deb: You wouldn't plan yours either?

Abby: No.

Deb: No?

Abby: I would just say, "Have a good time."

Deb: Have we done it? Have we done the interview?

Abby: I think we've done it. Is there anything else you'd like to say?

Deb: No. Just that it's been fun talking to you.

Abby: It's been a blast. Thank you, Deb. (Laughter.) I'm gonna have you sign a consent form.

Deb: Love to.